ISBN-13: 978-1480298569
ISBN-10: 1480298565

This study was funded by Alberta Innovates - Health Solutions, formerly the Alberta
Heritage Foundation for Medical Research, as part of the Preterm Birth and
Healthy Outcomes Team Interdisciplinary Team Grant (#200700595).

Research Team: Gerri C. Lasiuk, Jodi Jubinville, Kathy Hegadoren & Theirry Lacaze

Photographer: Emir Poelzer, Medical Photographer, Royal Alexandra Hospital,
Edmonton, AB

Writer/Designer: Laura Hanon

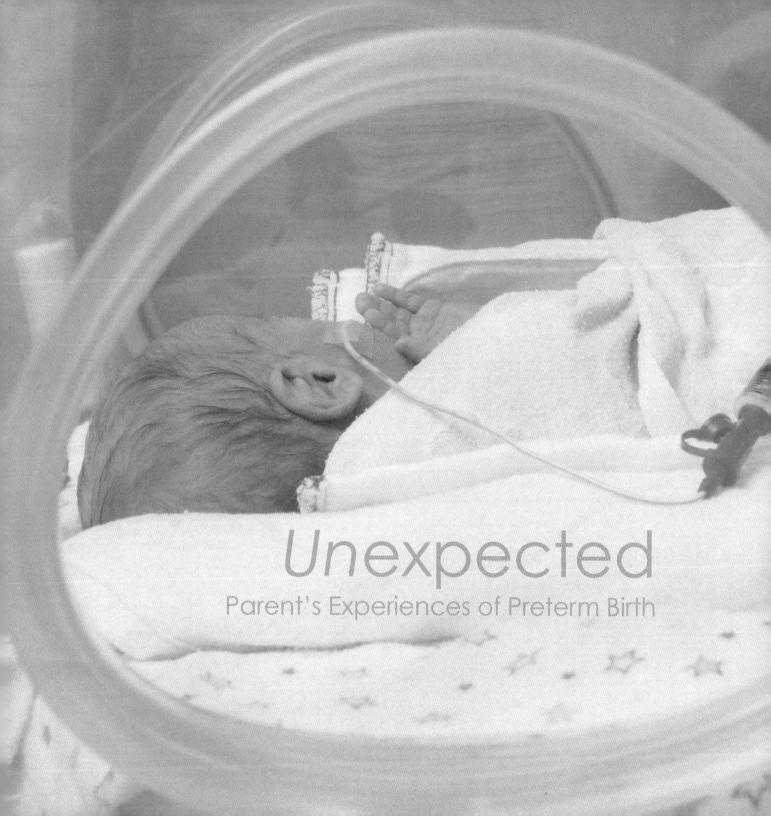

Unexpected
Parent's Experiences of Preterm Birth

Why Did We Write This Book?

Preterm birth catapults parents into the alien world of the Neonatal Intensive Care Unit (NICU), where the normalcy of everyday life fades and their only concern is their baby's precarious health. Often frightened and helpless, these parents are forced to rely on strangers to safeguard the life of their tiny baby who exists "betwixt the womb and the world."[1] As long as their infant remains medically fragile, uncertainty is high and even small changes can trigger new crises.

Recent research demonstrates that for many parents, having a preterm baby is a traumatic experience that shatters hopes and dreams of parenthood.

Humans use stories to organize and remember events in a coherent manner and to integrate thoughts and feelings into a meaningful whole. Traumatic events, like having a preterm baby, can disrupt these life stories.

In writing this book, we listened to parents' stories of having preterm babies and talked with some of the physicians, social workers, nurse practitioners, and nurses who work in the NICU.

From these conversations, we created and illustrated these stories. It is our hope that reading stories about preterm birth will help parents understand and manage their emotions and begin to rewrite their own life stories.

Gerri Lasiuk, RPN RN PhD
Certified Mental Health/Psychiatric Nurse (C)
Faculty of Nursing, University of Alberta

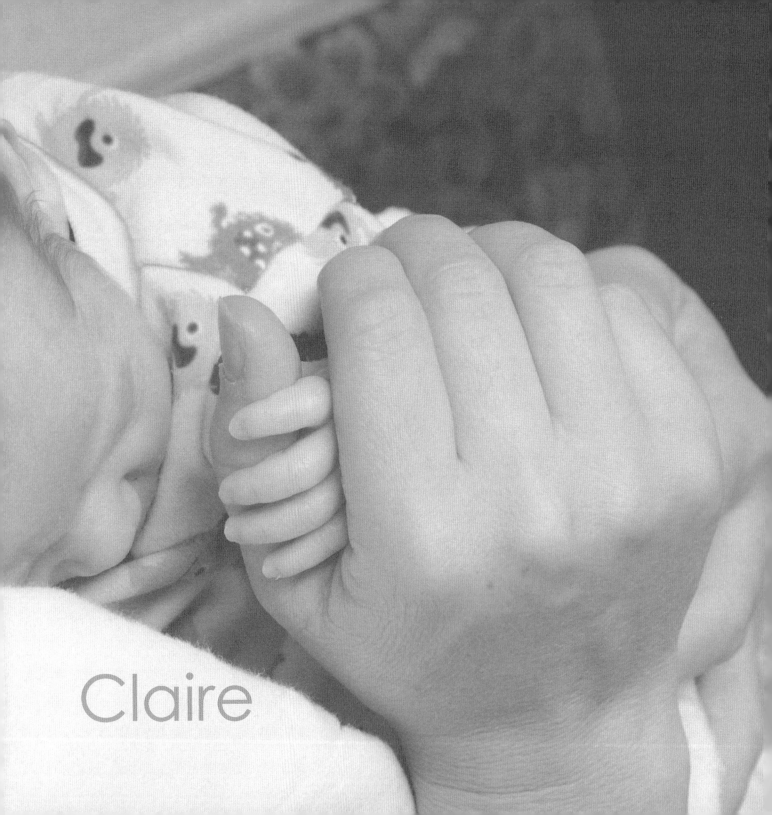

Claire

I first saw Anna sitting in her wheelchair next to the tiny incubator. She didn't move—just sat staring, wrapped in her housecoat. She reached her fingers toward the clear plastic, toward her infant and then drew them back. She turned to me, her face blank, her eyes wet.

I remember being in her place. The Neonatal Intensive Care Unit (NICU) seemed so foreign when I first walked in. There were rows of incubators and lots of machines that seemed smaller than they should be.

Called "pods," the individual rooms in the unit seemed at first like they belonged in some sort of spaceship. Infants were hidden in the incubators under quilts to mute the light. I remember bringing a baby quilt from home to place on top. Even if I couldn't wrap my newborn in it, at least he could have it close by.

The first time I saw my son Matthew, I felt like I was looking at an alien. His skin was transparent and the tiny blue veins looked as if they were painted on the surface. He had a breathing mask that covered most of his face, wires attached to his chest and fine tubes in his arms. I was terrified. I had been expecting a normal delivery like with my first child.

When Sarah was born, I went to the hospital when my water broke two days

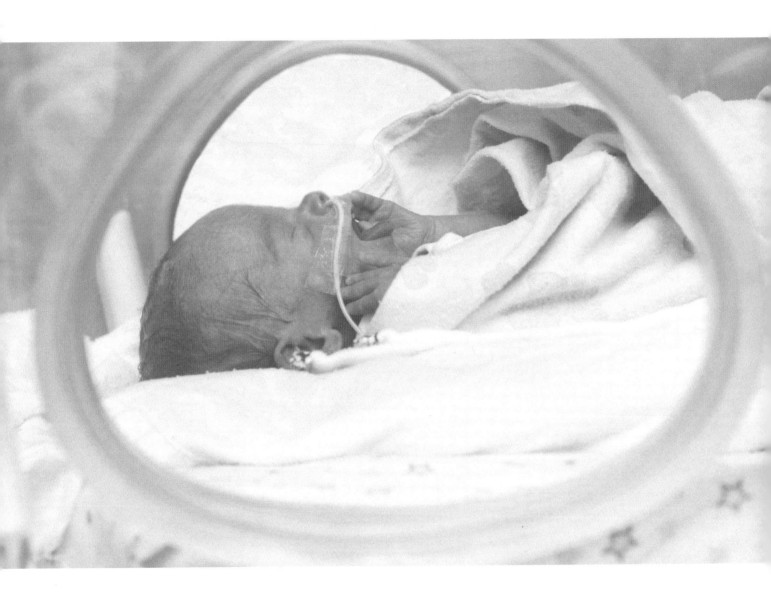

before my due date.

I cursed my husband as I endured painful labour.

I begged for and received an epidural.

Sarah was born.

I held her for the first time.

A nurse watched to make sure she latched on during breastfeeding and then we went home even, it seemed at the time, before people had finished visiting and bringing baby gifts.

With Matthew, it was different. I was shocked to find myself in a situation I didn't expect. From the moment I went into labour at 29 weeks, everything seemed surreal. At times it still does. But now at almost two months old, Matthew is still in the NICU and we are just waiting for him to pass the car seat test so we can take him home.

❧ ❧ ❧

Later that day, I saw Anna again—the woman from NICU. I had finished breastfeeding Matthew and was at the coffee shop in the food court of the hospital. This had become an informal gathering spot for NICU moms and sometimes dads and I was hoping to see some of the others there so we could catch up. Instead I saw her, still in her housecoat, sitting in a

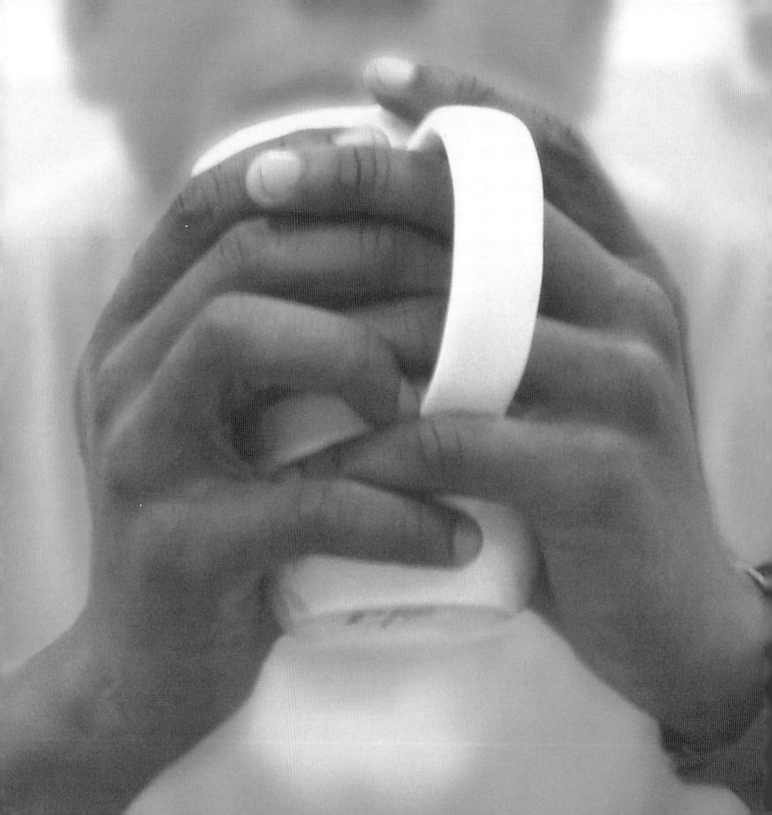

wheelchair pulled up to a table. She grasped an extra large cup with the tag from a tea bag hanging over the edge.

Where was her husband? Why was she there alone?

I ordered a decaf coffee and treated myself to a donut with the sprinkles. Matthew had gained another ounce and I was celebrating. I stopped by her table.

"Let me guess," I said. "Herbal tea?"

She looked at me but didn't answer. She seemed shell-shocked.

"I saw you in the NICU when I was visiting my son Matthew. My son was in that pod after he was born."

She looked at me then—really looked at me.

"I don't know what to do," she said. "I just had to get out of there for a while…"

I understood. I sat down and touched her arm gently as she set her tea down on the table.

"I'm Claire," I said. "Isn't there anyone here with you?"

She shook her head. "I live out of town. My husband was here but he had to

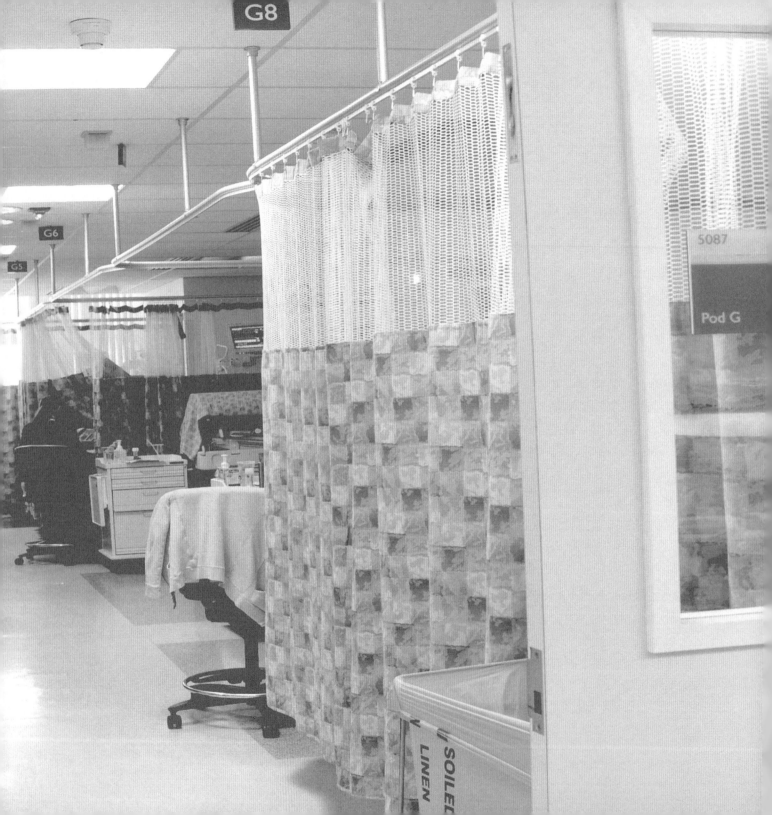

go back to work. He runs his own business and is trying to find someone to fill in, but it's hard…He'll be back on the weekend."

I didn't know what to do…so I started to talk.

"C-section?" I asked gesturing toward the wheelchair.

She nodded.

"I'm surprised you're out of bed."

"I just don't want to be here at all," she said. "I wasn't supposed to deliver for another two months."

She picked up her tea, but didn't drink it.

"I think everyone feels like that at the beginning. It's just scary. And it's horrible because you don't know what's going on," I said. "Is this your first child?"

She nodded and a tear rolled down her cheek. "It was supposed to be perfect."

I nodded. I thought my second delivery would be perfect too. I didn't expect to be spending every waking minute in the NICU, sleep deprived and feeling guilty for not spending enough time with Sarah or my husband. But, I was lucky. I had an extended family to help look after my first child and

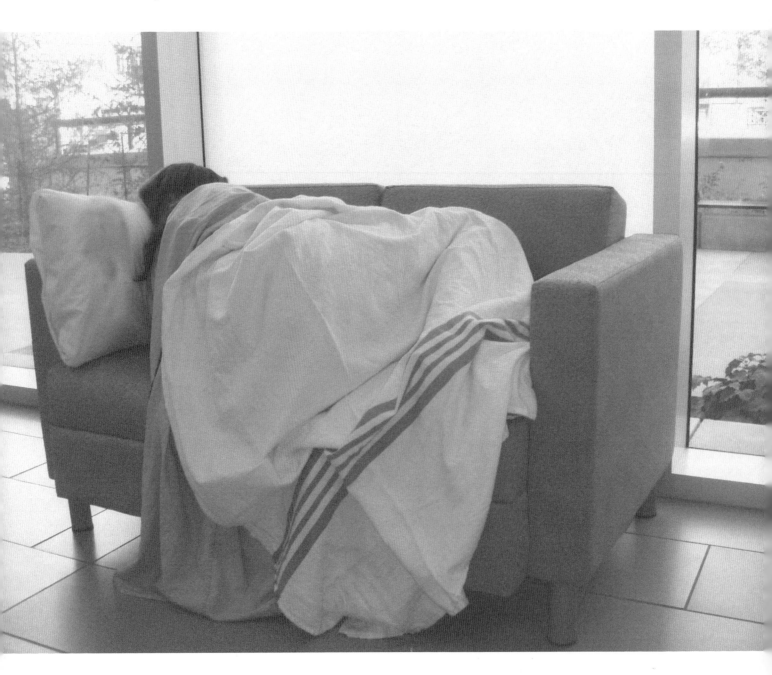

my husband came to the hospital every night after work. Now that I knew Matthew was coming home soon, I was starting to get excited—but not too excited. I didn't want to jinx anything.

I looked at my watch. I needed to get back upstairs to be with Matthew, I didn't like to leave him alone too long, but I couldn't leave this woman alone either.

"Why don't you show me your baby?" I asked.

She nodded and slowly wheeled toward the elevator as I followed.

❧ ❧ ❧

Anna's daughter was in the pod for the sickest preterm babies. The lights were dim; the room was warm; and there was a noise monitor on the wall as a polite reminder to keep the sound levels low. The lights of the monitor stayed green if the area was quiet but turned red if the noises rose higher than a whisper. I wheeled the woman over to her baby's incubator.

"There you are Anna," a nurse whispered as we entered the room. It was one of the nurses I knew well and I nodded to her.

"Your baby's doing just fine," the nurse said. "Have you picked a name for her yet?"

Anna shook her head.

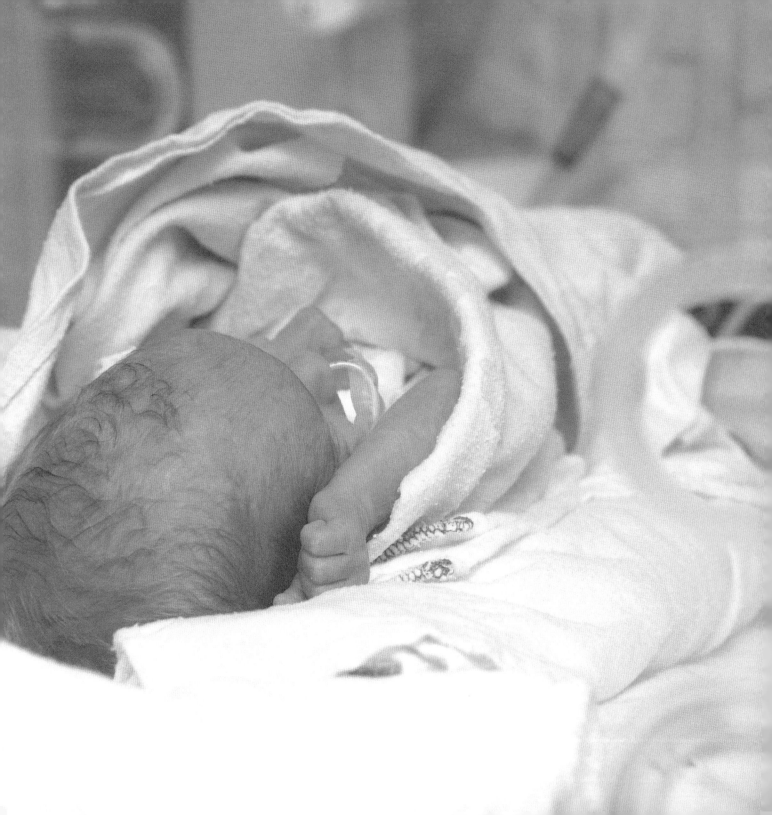

"Now, I think the doctor explained that we gave her surfactant to help her lungs and to make it easier for her to breathe. Do you have any questions?"

Anna shook her head again.

I looked at my watch. I was tired and it was time to feed Matthew again. I had to make sure there was enough breast milk in the fridge for the nighttime feedings. If not, I would be pumping more. If there weren't enough machines for the babies in this place already, there was one for the mothers as well— the dratted breast pump.

"What are all these things attached to her?" Anna asked the nurse.

"We went over them a few hours ago," The nurse responded. I knew that it was about time for shift change but she patiently went through each tube and each machine, explaining what it did and why it was there.

"The tube in her mouth is a breathing tube because she can't breathe on her own yet. Those round things on her chest are to monitor her heart…"

⚘ ⚘ ⚘

The next day, Anna came to find me as I was breastfeeding Matthew. It was his eight a.m. feeding. One time, I was a little late and was annoyed to find a nurse bottle-feeding formula to Matthew. She said that she hadn't been able to find the breast milk I had stored in the fridge. I know I stored extra milk in the freezer. I don't think she bothered to look there.

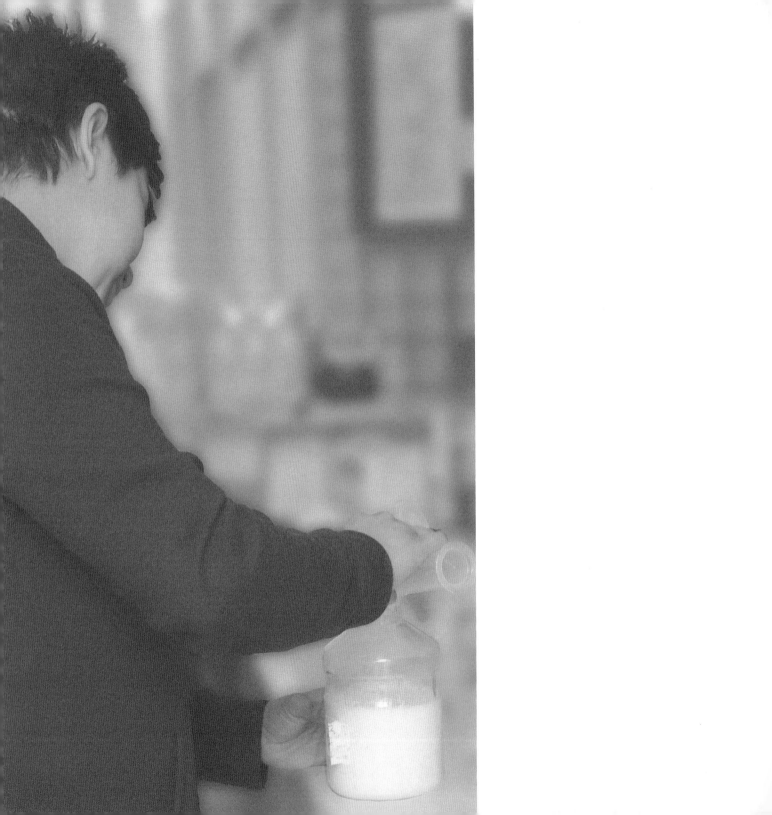

It wasn't a big deal to her but it certainly was to me. I remember crying for almost an hour. I felt robbed. Breastfeeding was the only thing I could do for my baby at that time. So many things were out of my control, but at least I could provide breast milk for Matthew. After that incident, I just always made sure to be at the hospital for the first feeding and I put a big note in his area that read: Breast milk in the fridge.

Anna sat with me a while and then we went down for coffee. It was impossible to talk in the unit. It was so important to keep a quiet environment for the babies.

"I don't know what I would do if this was my first child," I said to Anna.

"How many weeks were you?" she asked.

"29," I said. "I went home after work—I'm a teacher—and I just started to cramp a little. I thought they were Braxton Hicks contractions like I had with my daughter."

"I never had those. I don't even know what those are," Anna said.

"Oh, those are just 'pretend contractions' or false labour. A lot of women get them. Only mine never went away. They just got stronger and I became frightened. Then I went to the bathroom and there was blood everywhere. I freaked out. My daughter was crying because she was scared I was dying. I couldn't get a hold of my husband, so I called an ambulance to take us both to the hospital. My daughter still has nightmares about it."

Unexpected

"… you shut down essentially… we hit a point where both of us were just in total and utter shock. We didn't know what to do, what to say…it's like you're in this really messed up dream and everything's moving faster than you can comprehend it."

—Father of a preterm baby

"(It was) all very surreal… it all happened very fast and very slow at the same time … he needed some help breathing… (and) he got taken away pretty quickly… I actually didn't get to see him. I don't remember seeing him."

—Mother of a preterm baby

I paused for a moment. I didn't expect it would be so painful to retell this story.

"When they saw all the blood in Emergency, they whisked me in pretty quickly. I remember thinking that if I squeezed my legs together really tightly, I could stop everything from happening. I didn't even want to let the doctor examine me."

"I get it," Anna said. "I was on bed rest at home for three weeks before coming here. They were trying to stop me from going into labour. My husband would go to work every day and leave a sandwich and a bottle of water by the bed. I stared at the ceiling for weeks."

"Three weeks! I would have gone nuts. All you can think about is doing everything possible to not have the baby, right?"

"Right…that and the water stain on the ceiling," she said absently. "I stared at that stain for hours…and worried about everything that could go wrong. I had to get up to go to the bathroom though. I think that's why my baby was born early."

"It's not your fault," I said. "Most of the time, nobody knows why women go into labour early. I didn't have any of the medical problems that can cause premature labour. And I didn't smoke or take drugs so those things weren't factors."

I took a sip of coffee.

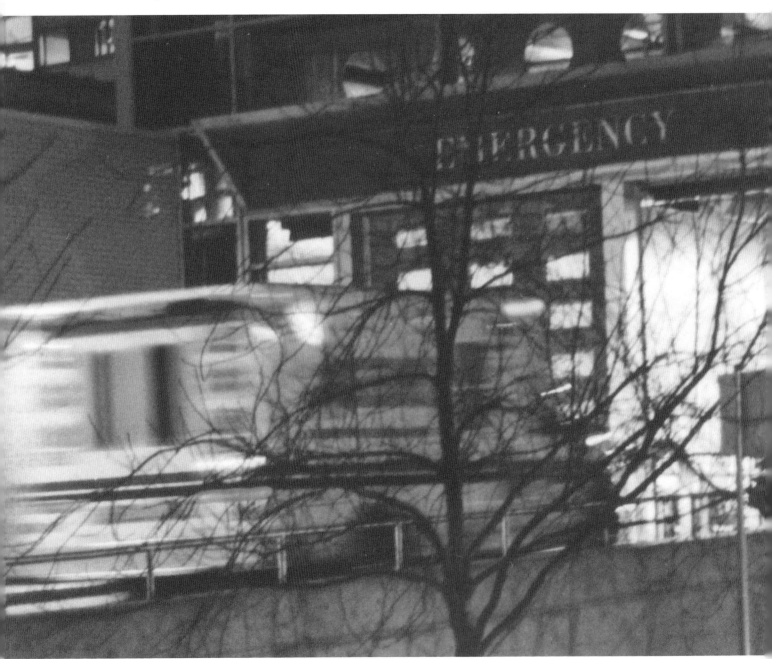

"No one knows why I went into labour early," I said. "I was terrified. I didn't even know if a baby that little would live. Some doctor—a resident I think—came in and told me all the things that could go wrong with a 29-week-old baby.

"My husband Tom wasn't there because he was trying to hand off our daughter Sarah to his mom. This doctor was so impersonal and clinical. He didn't seem to realize that this was the worst thing that had ever happened to me—to us. That this was my *baby* he was talking about. I wanted to cover my ears and yell at him to stop as he listed everything that could go wrong.

"After I delivered Matthew they took him away before I could even see him. He was a breach delivery. I didn't even hear him crying so I didn't know if he was dead or alive. My husband didn't know whether to stay with me or go with Matthew to the NICU. I told him to go, *go.* I couldn't stand thinking of our tiny baby all alone. I remember being terrified because I didn't know what was happening with Matthew for a very long time.

"Finally Tom came back and told me Matthew was alive, but that he was really sick."

I took a sip of my decaf coffee. Anna looked pale. She looked overloaded.

"Are you okay?" I asked.

She nodded, but then started to sob. Big fat tears rolled down her face in the middle of the food court. I wanted to tell her that her baby would be okay, but

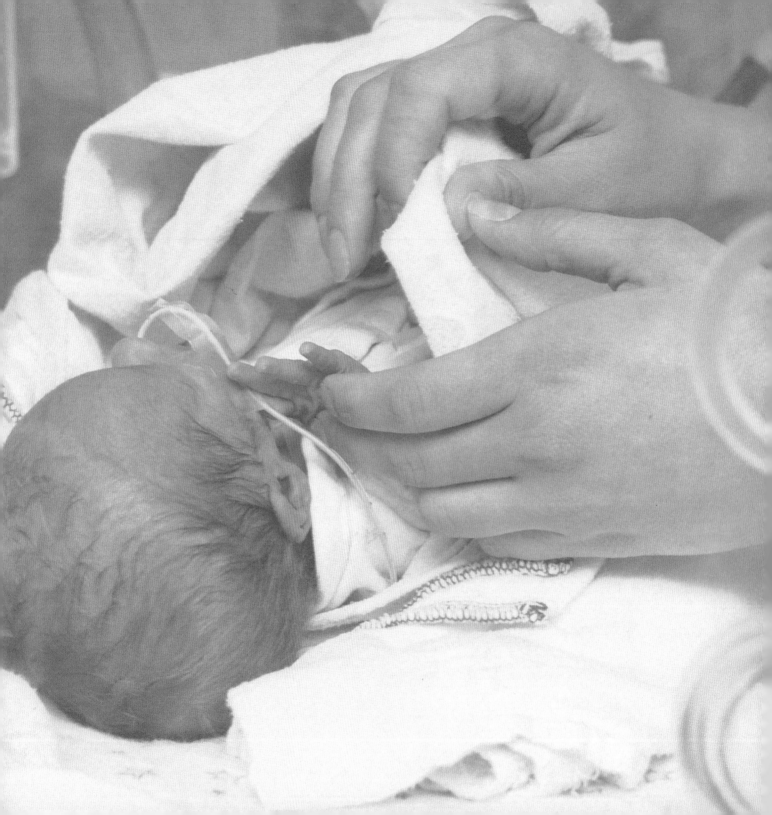

I couldn't. Nobody could.

"I don't know how you do it," she said. "I just don't know what I'm supposed to be doing or what I'm allowed to do…"

"Listen," I said. "This is your baby. I know it's hard, but you need to find out everything you can about her condition every day. Go to morning rounds and ask the doctors and other staff questions."

"I don't know what to ask," she said, "and I can't remember things that they tell me."

I stopped for a minute and thought. How would she know? She'd never had a child before. I tried to remember back to when Matthew was first born. It seemed so long ago. I remember how overwhelmed I felt. I had my husband for support. She had nobody.

"Okay," I said. "Do you have a notebook?"

She shook her head.

"One way you can remember things is to write them down. I know that you don't feel like it right now, but it might help to remember things and to know what to ask.

"Another thing that helped me was to talk to the nurses. Ask them to explain things to you that you don't understand. It doesn't matter if you forget and

Unexpected

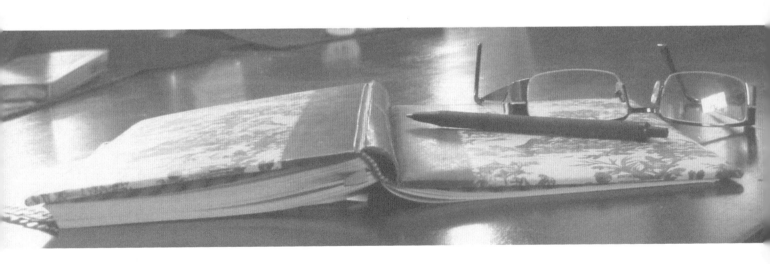

have to ask again. They're used to it. The thing you have to understand is that every parent who comes into the NICU has no idea what to do or what's going on. This is a hard thing to deal with, but you're her mother and she needs you."

Poor Anna, I thought. She looked lost. But, I had my own responsibilities. I needed to call Sarah at my mom's and it was just about time for Matthew's next feeding.

"Have you met the social worker yet?" I asked.

Anna shook her head.

Then I saw some other NICU moms come over to our table. We had all become close in the last few weeks. It was a comfort to talk to moms who knew what I was going through.

"Anna, this is Preeti and Joy."

Preeti adjusted her hijab (head scarf) as she sat down. The women introduced themselves and they began to talk.

"Anna, I have to go feed Matthew now. Talk to you later, okay?"

She nodded and I headed up the stairs.

It was always like this, I thought. Rushing from one thing to another—always

"… I also felt like that it was all my fault and … I felt a grieving that I couldn't mother him the way that I would if we coulda taken him home that, the next day… I wasn't doing my job properly and (I felt) inadequate knowing that—as a woman—I was not capable of doing it the way everyone should do it."

—Mother of a preterm baby

"… I think it was almost at the two-week mark. It was 4 in the morning and my husband and I were in the NICU and I'm just like 'I need you to take me home right now!'… I hadn't slept in a long time and my doctor had given me Xanax to help me sleep."

—Mother of a preterm baby

on a schedule. Finally though, I had hope. There hadn't been any for so long.

Matthew seemed to have every problem a preemie could have. He was jaundiced; couldn't breathe on his own; and couldn't eat except through a feeding tube. I sat beside him for days as they took blood, monitored his heart rate and stuck an IV tube in his head. That was the worst thing to see. All I could think of was the pain he felt every time they stuck something into him.

The social worker helped me to see that the nursing staff was doing things *for* him and not *to* him. Looking at it that way helped me each time I watched a new procedure.

The scariest thing for us was that Matthew's lungs weren't working properly. He just couldn't breathe on his own and had a breathing tube in for a long time. I remember thinking that he must barely be alive if he couldn't breathe.

I expected the doctors and nurses to know what was wrong and fix it. It took me a while to realize that sometimes they just don't know. They do tests and monitor your baby, but they have no magic fixes. I was expecting to be told, your baby has *a*, *b* and *c* and we need to do *this*, *this* and *this* to fix it… just like when you have a cold or flu, but it's not like that at all. Not at all.

When I reached Matthew's pod, I washed my hands and picked him up. He was such a fighter. I stroked his head and set him down to change his diaper. Then I washed my hands again and settled down to breastfeed. I stared at him as he suckled and was filled with joy and love for him.

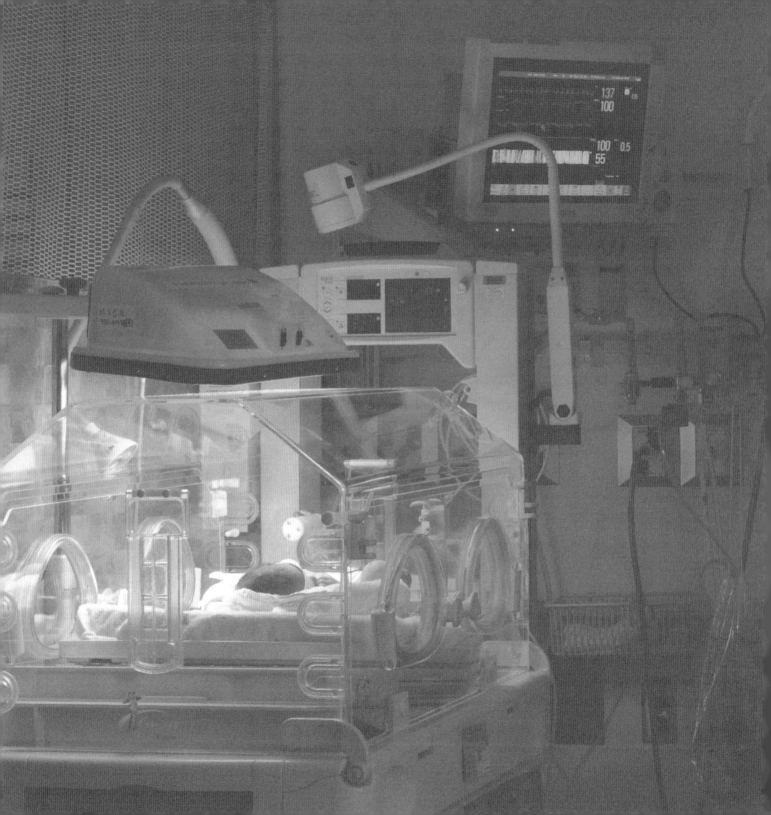

I didn't always feel that love. When I was at Anna's stage—shell-shocked—I couldn't bond with Matthew at all. I wanted to see him so badly after he was born, but then when I did, I felt nothing. Absolutely nothing. I didn't even think he was my baby. He looked so strange. I was afraid to touch him. Where do you put your hand when there are so many wires attached to that little body? What if I accidently pulled some out? The nurse told me to cradle him by cupping my hand around him like a hug because his skin was so delicate and my first thought was, *Where*? I didn't want to look like a bad mother, so I tried and then pulled away.

Looking back, I think that it was hard for me to bond with Matthew because I wasn't sure he was going to live. I didn't want to fall in love with him and then lose him. My main concern was to do everything to keep him alive, but now I resent not being able to bond with him right away.

I often thought that I was a bad mother because I didn't feel anything for my own child, but I know now that the inability to bond has nothing to do with being a good or bad mother. It has to do with simply being human.

As Matthew suckled, I thought of Sarah sitting at home with my mom. I feel so guilty not being able to be with her. Until Matthew's birth we'd spent so much time together. We'd talked about her new brother or sister and she'd been so excited. Now I have to divide my time between the two of them and find that I spend most of my time at the hospital. Sarah understands as much as any four-year-old can, but I know she misses me and we'll never get this time back.

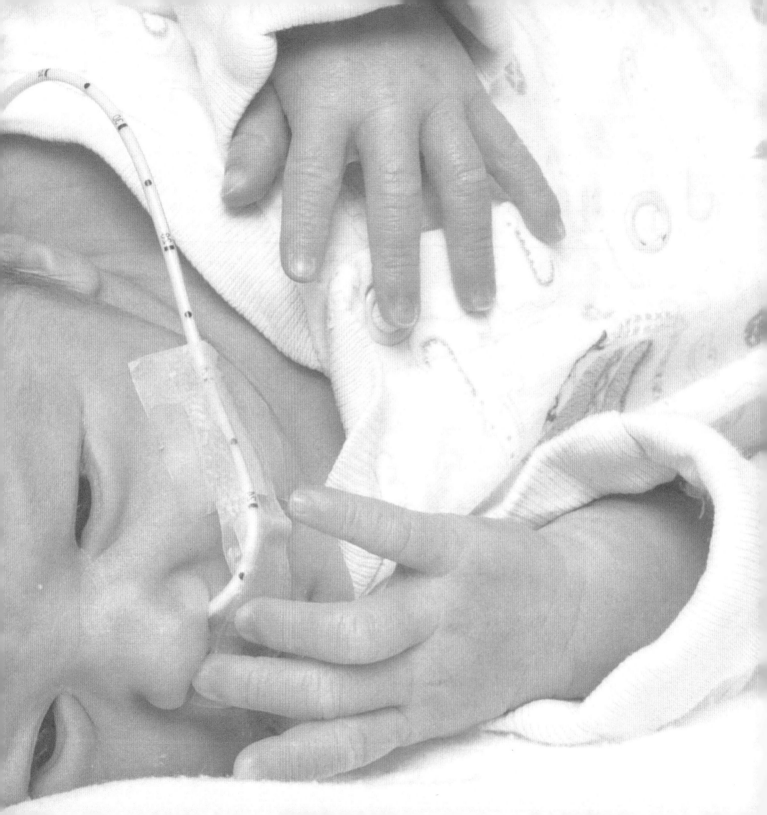

I know from talking to other moms that we're lucky she can stay with family members. What do other parents do if they don't have family support? I can't imagine not being able to spend time with Matthew because I had to look after Sarah. And what if I lived out of town and could only see him on the weekends? Our family's been through a lot, but I know that things are much tougher for other families.

After I fed Matthew, I cuddled with him and then chatted with the nurses before my husband Tom showed up. He usually dropped by after work and stayed a few hours.

I usually left about seven or eight, picked Sarah up and spent some time with her before putting her to bed. It meant that she went to bed later than she should, but for now it was what worked for our family. The only time Tom and I spent together was when we were with Matthew. He stayed after I left, fed Matthew his bottle and headed home around 10 or 11.

Tom walked over. The nurses greeted him as he arrived.

"How's Matthew?" he asked me.

It was what he always asked. He never asked how I was any more. Everything was centered on Matthew. I knew what was coming. He would ask for the details. How many times did he poop? How long did he breastfeed? How many hours did he sleep? Then he would record everything on his laptop.

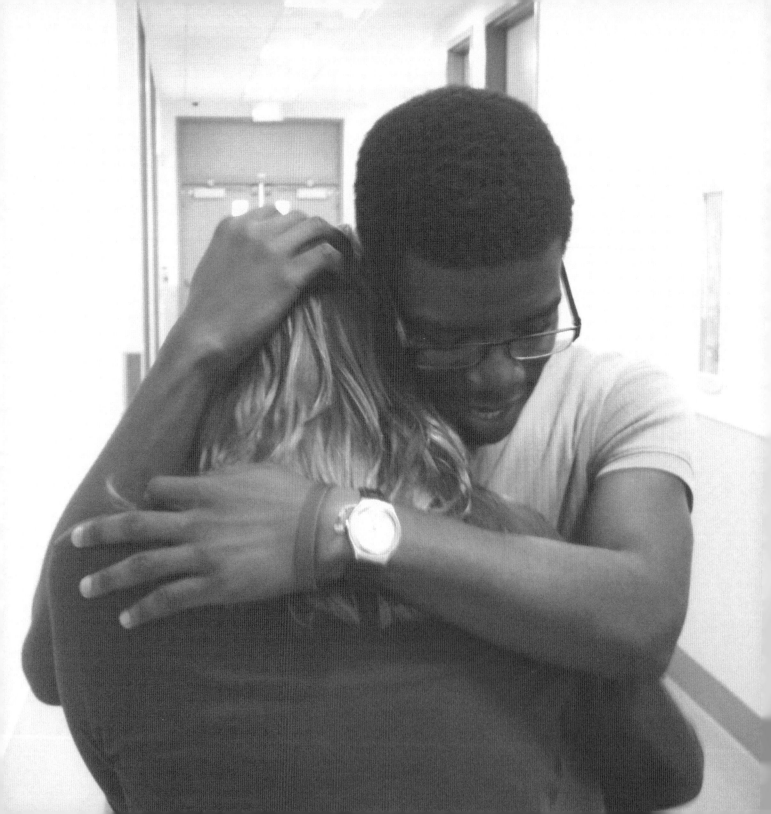

"Good," I said.

I filled him in on the day and watched as he studiously recorded everything. I know keeping track of these details helped him feel like he was doing something, but what I really wanted was for him to ask me how I was. How *I* was feeling.

One of the nurses came for the daily weigh-in. This was the highlight of Tom's day and he tried never to miss it. As Matthew's weight was recorded, Tom peppered the nurse with questions. Matthew had gained an ounce. What did that mean? Could Matthew go home early? All the nurses were used to Tom's questions and she answered him patiently.

I suppose I should feel fortunate. A lot of husbands don't spend much time in the NICU. Sometimes they just can't because of work or other obligations and sometimes I think they just feel out of place—like they aren't needed.

Anna's husband wouldn't be able to come at all until the weekend. I just wish that Tom wasn't so obsessed with the baby. I had been through a lot too and I needed him sometimes just to hold me and tell me that everything was going to be all right.

Unexpected

"... if I didn't have (my mom) I don't know what I would have done... she brought me food to the hospital so that I wouldn't have to eat the hospital food... [and] they drove us everywhere, even after (our daughter) came out of the hospital."

—Mother of a preterm baby

"... my brother-in-law went up with me to the NICU and... it was good to have him there because I pretty much fell on my knees... it was very, very scary..."

—Father of a preterm baby

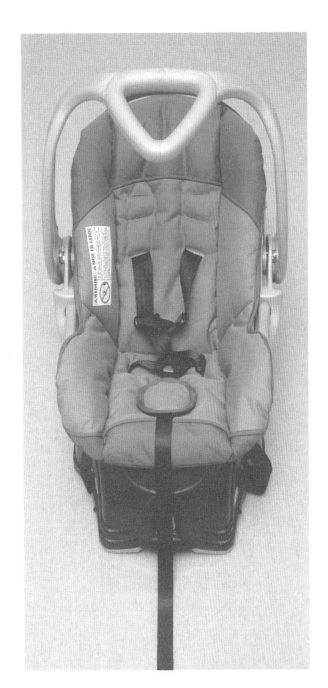

Tom

I don't get it. I never seem to do anything right. When I saw Claire today, she seemed pissed off again. She spends every waking minute at the hospital with Matthew. I get that she's worried, but she barely talks to me any more. She doesn't want to listen when I show her Matthew's growth chart on my computer or my projections about his potential release date.

She never bothered to learn the names of the machines that once kept our son alive. She just nick-named them—breathing box, heart-beater, feed-tube thingie. She even called the incubator the glass coffin for the first few days—even though it was made out of plastic.

The first thing I do when I get to the unit is check Matthew's chart. Then I talk to Claire and the nurses to see what happened during his day. I can't be there for morning rounds so I listen to the daily recording I've asked Claire to make. That way I can hear directly what was said. I snap the daily picture on my phone and forward it to my Facebook page so everyone can see how he's doing.

Some days I envy Claire because she can spend all day here. I can't. I have to work or we won't eat. We'll lose the house. It took all of our savings to buy the house just after we had our daughter. We knew it would be tight for a few years, but we needed the room and weren't expecting this.

"In the beginning it was very, very taxing and very stressful and very hard on us and, uh, tested a lot of things about our, our marriage and finances and everything."
—Father of a preterm baby

"… my wife and I have been married 6 years and we really hadn't gone through anything… a hardship together … so to go through something together that affects you so much emotionally, uhm, and you kinda learn how to, how to support each other… now I think we know each other better…"
—Father of a preterm baby

I took a few weeks off work at the beginning when Matthew was really ill, but we needed my full salary to cover our bills. I even had to put in a little overtime to make up the time I lost.

Still we are better off than some families. We met a young couple who don't have a car and have to bus here from the other end of the city. I think the social worker told them they could get discounted bus passes but even so…

The mom brings her lunch and dinner from home every day. She told me she can't afford to buy food here. One day, someone accidently (or on purpose) took her food from the fridge and she had nothing to eat all day. Who would do that? When Claire found out, she bought her some soup. And it turns out their baby probably has vision and hearing problems. We're lucky compared to them. Matthew was sick for a while, but now he's almost ready to go home.

The hospital staff has been great for the most part, but it seems sometimes they could be more efficient. Like when Matthew had to go for his hernia operation. Hernias are pretty common for preemie boys but the operation was done in another hospital. We only had an hour's notice before he was transferred over there. Claire found out by cell phone on a rare occasion when she'd left the hospital in the middle of the day to spend time with our daughter, Sarah. She dropped Sarah off at my mom's and raced over to the other hospital. Now she won't leave the hospital at all. It's like if she stays here, nothing bad will happen.

I left work and met her there. It was a whole new place. Everything was different. We couldn't find parking. When we did, it was outrageously expensive. At least at this hospital, we have a reduced-rate parking pass.

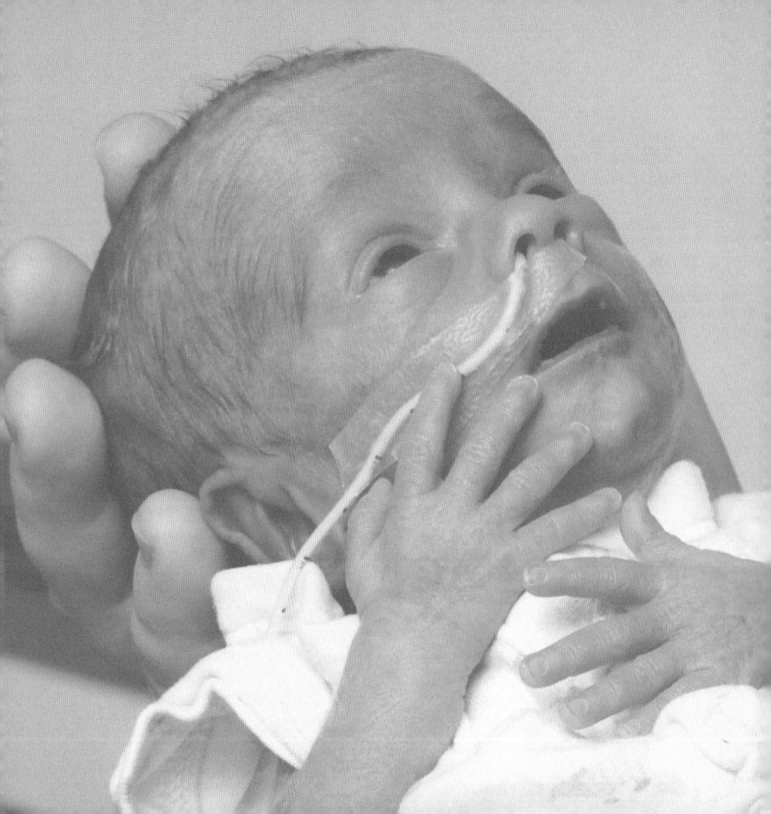

Then we had no idea where we were going. When we finally found the right unit, they were already prepping Matthew for surgery and we couldn't even see him. He's our baby, right? It felt like the doctors and nurses were taking over our baby. It wasn't as if this was emergency surgery or a life or death situation.

Claire was devastated. Fortunately the nurses there were really good. They explained that when a bed opens up for surgery, things happen quickly. Transfers don't usually happen with such little notice, but when a bed is open they have to act.

Of course we wanted Matthew to have the surgery and were happy he was there, but we were left emotionally raw. Hadn't we been through enough already? It took us both a few hours to calm down.

They also did things completely differently at the other hospital and they even used different terms. It's like I'd just learned a whole new language in the first NICU and now I needed to learn more new words. Why can't nurses call it breast milk? Why is it expressed breast milk or EBM?

Just when Claire was getting used to a routine at the second hospital they sent Matthew back here. That time we didn't even know he was being transferred. There was a mix-up with a new nurse on duty and she didn't call Claire to let her know what was happening. So Claire showed up at the hospital and there was no Matthew. She flipped out over that. The explanation was the same—a bed opened up and he was shipped back.

The thing that upset me is that moving Matthew back and forth set him back.

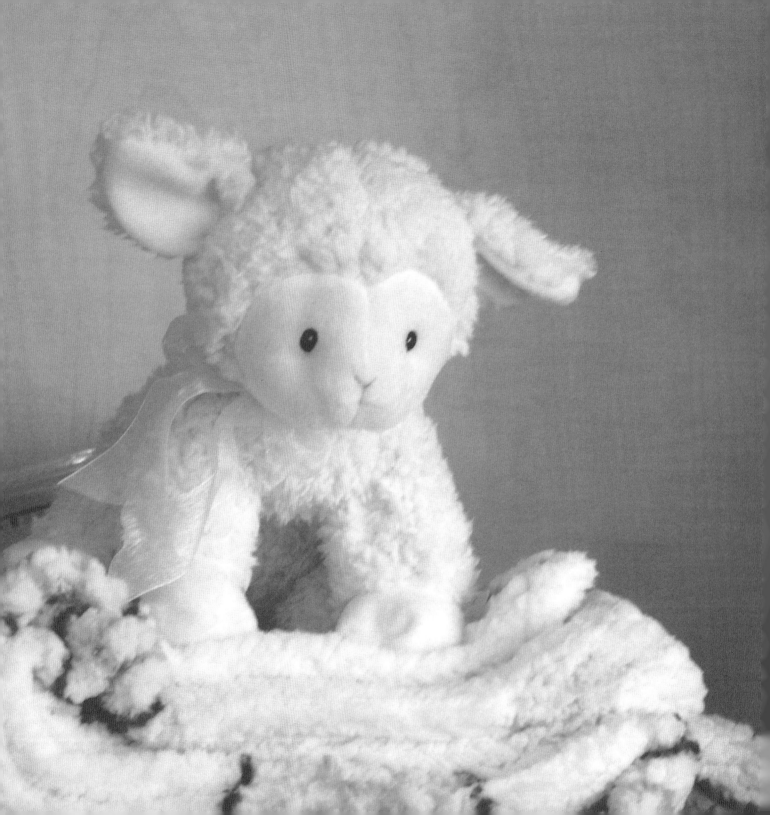

He had been gaining really well, but after the surgery and the transfers he lost a whole two ounces!

꿨 꿨 꿨

I have to say, it sometimes bothers me that Claire spends all of her time at the hospital. I race between work, home, here and Sarah. I get that she needs to be here, but I miss her. We're both exhausted and fighting more than usual.

I found her talking to her new friend, Anna.

"Claire, I need to talk to you," I said.

Claire raised her left eyebrow the way she always does when she thinks I'm going to ask for more facts about Matthew, but she excused herself from Anna and followed me to the hall.

"I want to ask you out to dinner."

"What? How can I do dinner with you when I can't even get home to see Sarah?"

"I just think it would be good for us," I said. "We could go across the road to that little restaurant and you can take your cell phone. We'll ask the nurses to call if they need you."

She rubbed her hands on her face. What, did I have to beg?

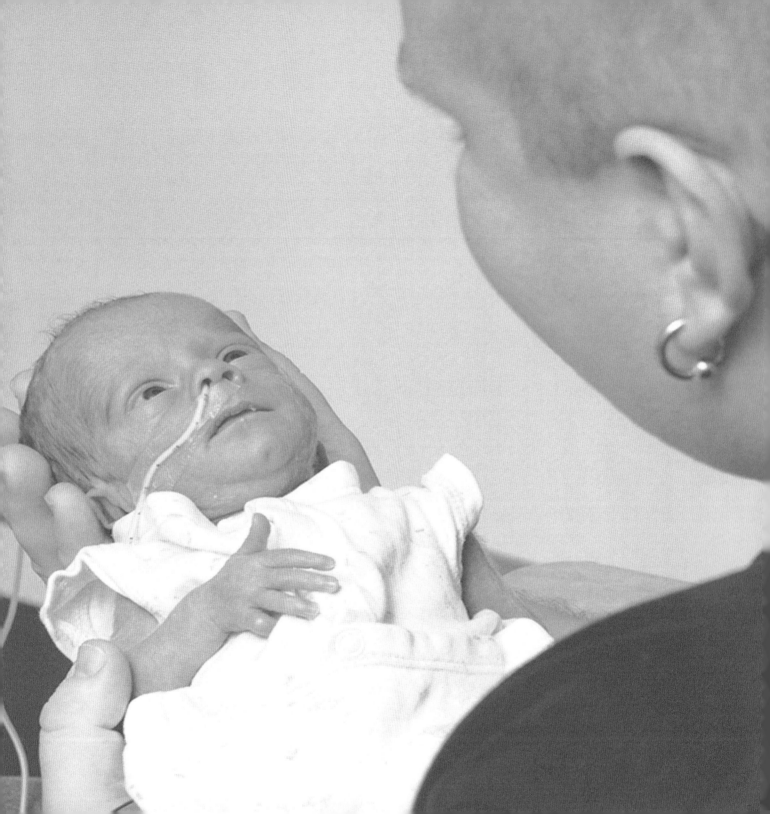

"We don't spend any time together anymore, Claire. We'll only be gone an hour."

"Like a date night?" she asked. When I nodded, she said, "Okay, but you can't bring your laptop, show me any of your charts or explain anything about Matthew to me."

"Deal," I said, "and I don't want to hear one word about breastfeeding."

Our date night went really well. We didn't talk about Matthew too much, but we did talk about the NICU almost the whole night. Since it had been the world we shared for the last few weeks, it seemed natural.

Claire did a funny impression of her favorite nurse and told me a truly inspiring story about a baby who initially had been given a five percent survival rate, but who had just left the hospital.

One of the interesting things we talked about was how people from different cultures and religions responded to things in the NICU. Claire and I weren't religious but I saw how one family had pulled through a really difficult week with the support of their pastor, family and lots of prayer. It really seemed to help them. I know the social worker at the hospital had offered great support and advice to another family we knew well.

"Hey, when we made any decisions about Matthew, we didn't really ask our parents or anyone else what we should do, right?" Claire asked.

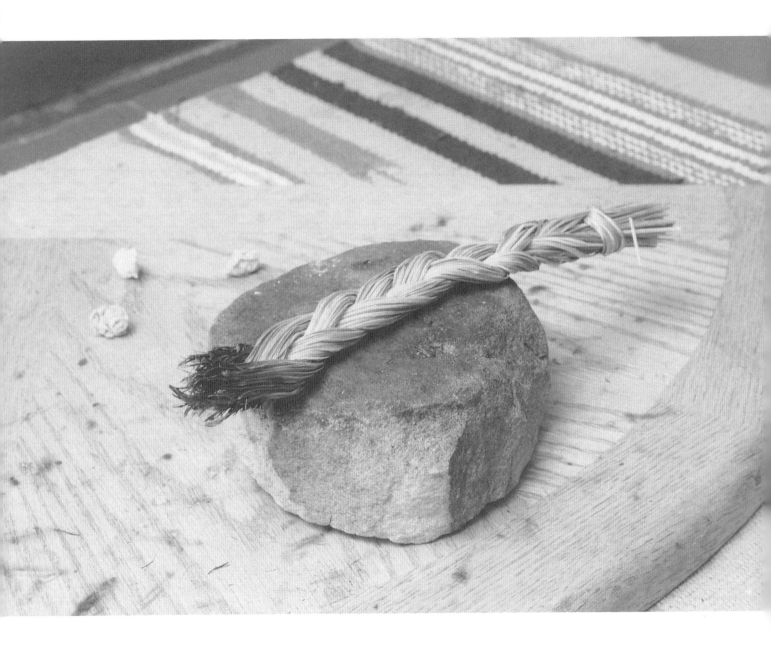

I nodded, "No, we pretty well decided on our own what to do."

"That's what I thought. Last week, I heard one family tell the nurse practitioner that they had to consult with their elders before deciding to proceed with a particular procedure. I thought it was so cool. And you know my friend Preeti?"

I nodded. Preeti was always at the hospital, but I had never seen her husband there.

"She has a huge extended family. They're going to help with her twins once they come home."

"That's good. I don't know what we would do without our parents to look after Sarah," I said. "Hey, how's your friend Anna coping?"

Claire shrugged. "It's hard to tell. Some days are better than others."

"Has she talked to the social worker yet?" I asked. "She looks like she's in shock most of the time."

"Give her a break. She's dealing with this all by herself."

"Claire, I'm not judging her. We know what it's like. It's just that I've been reading about acute stress disorder. It's pretty common in parents who have preterm births. Because we're taking Matthew home soon, I thought it was something we should be aware of after we leave the hospital, but maybe Anna should talk to someone about it now."

"… every day was different, you couldn't, you couldn't go in there expecting the same thing that happened yesterday or even a, a good step, `cause if you, if you went in expecting a weight gain and there was a weight loss it was just a complete downfall… you had to kind of pick yourself up again …"

—Mother of a preterm baby

"… having a baby in—in the NICU is that it really feels like a bit of a rollercoaster… at one moment in time it looks like things are getting better, and then your baby has a really bad night or your baby has a bad few hours … (it's) two steps forward (and) one step back."

—Mother of preterm baby

"What's wrong with Anna?"

"She just doesn't seem like she knows where she is half the time. Sometimes when I see her in the halls, she looks like she's sleepwalking—and I'm not the most observant guy. I only mention it, because you're friends and you might want to suggest she talk to someone about how she's doing."

Claire was looking at me like a protective lioness. I took a bite of my meal.

"So explain this acute stress disorder," she said.

"Well I've only been reading a little about it, but some people are affected by traumatic events—major crises like a car accident or serious illness—things that put you face-to-face with death. It's the same for us."

I paused.

"Remember when Matthew was born and we were absolutely terrified and felt helpless to do anything? I remember being on edge all the time. I read that some people have trouble concentrating and can have flashbacks or nightmares."

Claire leaned forward. "I remember being startled at the slightest thing. I was jumpy for weeks. But having a preterm birth is traumatic. Most of the parents I know have experienced all of those things."

"I know. Pretty much everyone who goes through a traumatic event is affected in some way. I read that it's a normal response to abnormal

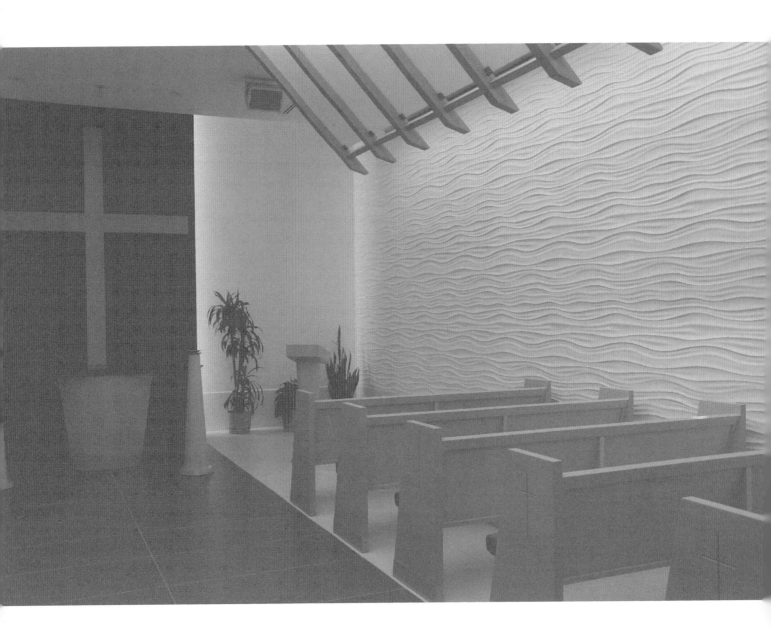

circumstances and that most people gradually get back to ... well, maybe not normal—you can never forget something like this—but they get much better. But, I read that if it goes on more than a month or so and the person can't function, it can turn into post-traumatic stress disorder. PTSD. Like war veterans."

I took a sip of my coffee. "You know Anna better than I do. I just thought I'd mention it."

Claire looked at me and for a minute she smiled at me the way she used to.

"It was really thoughtful of you to bring that up. I'll talk to Anna tomorrow."

She reached over and held my hand and for a moment I forgot everything but her.

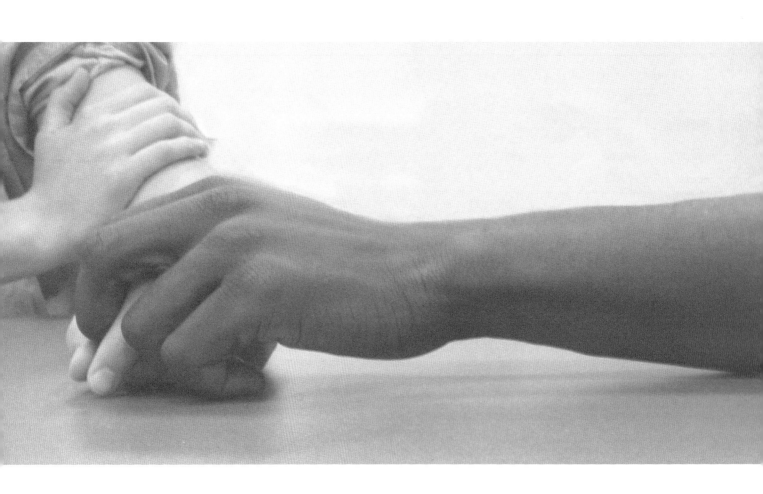

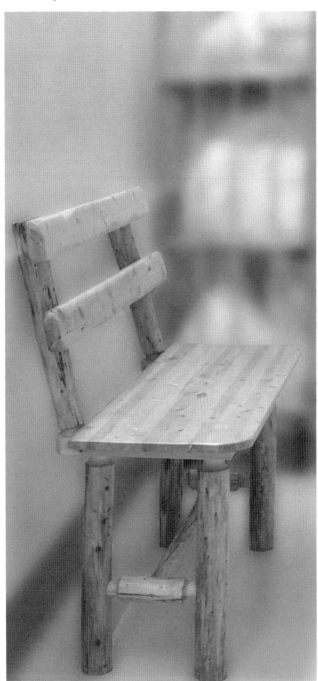

Anna

Claire is so strong. I don't know how she does it. Me, I'm just scared all the time. I can't eat and I'm barely sleeping. When I do doze off for a few minutes, I wake up shaking and terrified. Mostly, I don't understand what's going on. It's not the nurses' faults. They keep explaining things over and over but I just can't seem to grasp the simplest things right now. I don't even know what the nurses and doctors are talking about half the time. It's like they're speaking a foreign language.

I'm not used to babies. I never babysat and don't even know how to diaper a normal baby. How am I supposed to diaper a baby the size of my hand? The nurses tell me to touch her and talk to her, but I'm too afraid.

I wish my husband was here but he's at home, up north, trying to keep the business going. He's going to drive down on the weekend, but it's so hard not having him here.

We haven't even chosen a name for our baby yet. Every night on the phone, I try to tell him what the doctors have said, but it's hard to remember. Claire told me to keep a journal and make a list of the questions I want to ask. She even bought me a small notebook from the dollar store and brought it in because I didn't have a vehicle to get around. Since I started recording things, it's been easier to give the information to my husband.

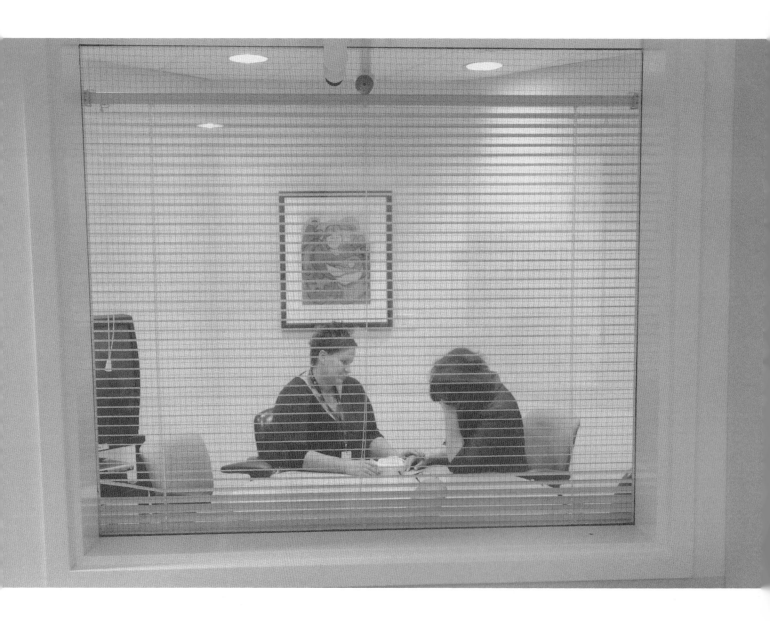

I wrote in my journal that the baby had jaundice and was placed under a light to get rid of it. That night on the phone, I could explain it to my husband and that made me feel good.

The first time I saw the baby, I didn't know what to think. She didn't look real. There was a tube coming out of her head that freaked me out. It turned out to be an IV like the one I had in my arm during the C-section. I don't know why they put it in her head. Maybe Claire will know.

My baby's also on this thing called CPAP to help her breathe. I think that's better than the breathing tube she had before but I'm not sure. I wrote it in my journal so I can ask a nurse at rounds tomorrow.

The social worker, Janice, came to see me yesterday. I can't remember half of what she said. I can't seem to focus on anything. When I talked to Claire about the visit, she told me to go back to see Janice today—she even came with me. I think she's worried about me. I am worried about me too. What if I'm going crazy? Claire and I talked with Janice about different ways to handle the stress of being in the NICU.

When Janice told us that it's normal to feel anxious or depressed, I burst into tears. It felt good to finally tell someone that most days I don't want to get out of bed and I have to force myself to dress. I haven't put on clean clothes for days and I can't remember when I took my last shower. Claire hugged me and then we both ended up laughing when she said hasn't shaved her legs in weeks.

After that, I made a list in my journal of all the things I can think of to look

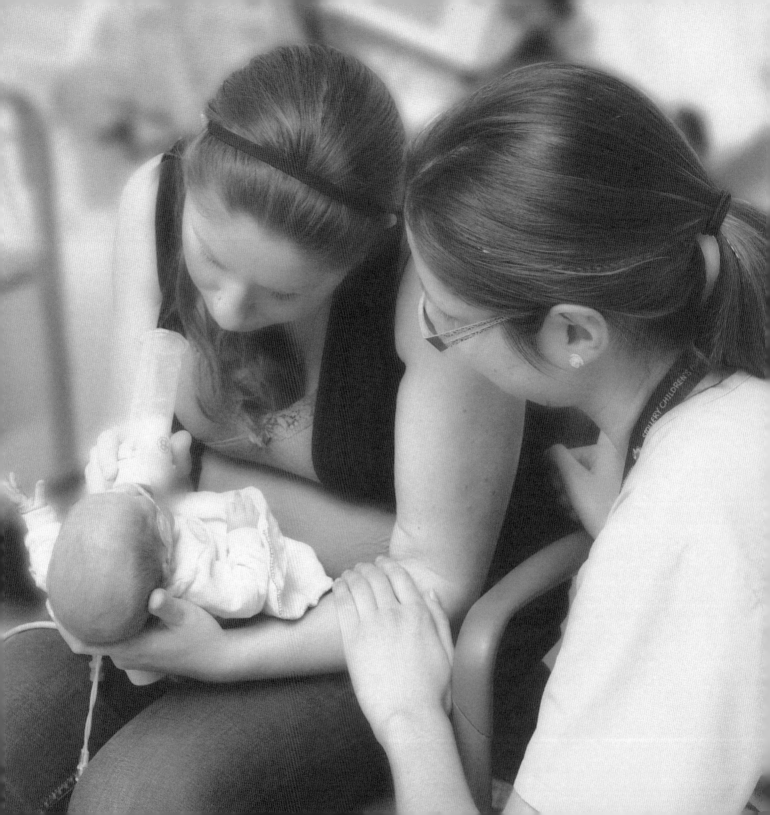

after myself.

My list is pretty simple.

1. Try to eat something every two hours.
2. Lie down and relax for 30 minutes every four hours. (I might even try a relaxation DVD.)
3. Go for two walks every day.

At least now I know I'm not losing it. Janice said that everyone handles the stress of having a baby in the NICU in different ways and that it might help if I talked to some of the other moms to see how they're coping. I think I might even make an appointment with my family doctor to see if there's anything else I can do.

Talking about things really helped. There's a really nice nurse who talks to me a lot about what is going on. If I didn't have her and Claire, I don't know if I would make it through this. I'm starting to meet some of the other moms and just hearing their stories helps a lot. I'm just so shy; it's hard for me to reach out for help.

The baby beside mine cries all the time. The nurse told me that the mother was addicted to drugs and that the baby will be given up for adoption or put in foster care when she is well enough. This baby has a different type of cry than mine and sometimes I am barely able to stay in the room. She just keeps crying and crying this pitiful sound that tears at my heart. Then I think that all she has are the nurses to care for her. She has no one to love her yet and that helps me get through the constant crying.

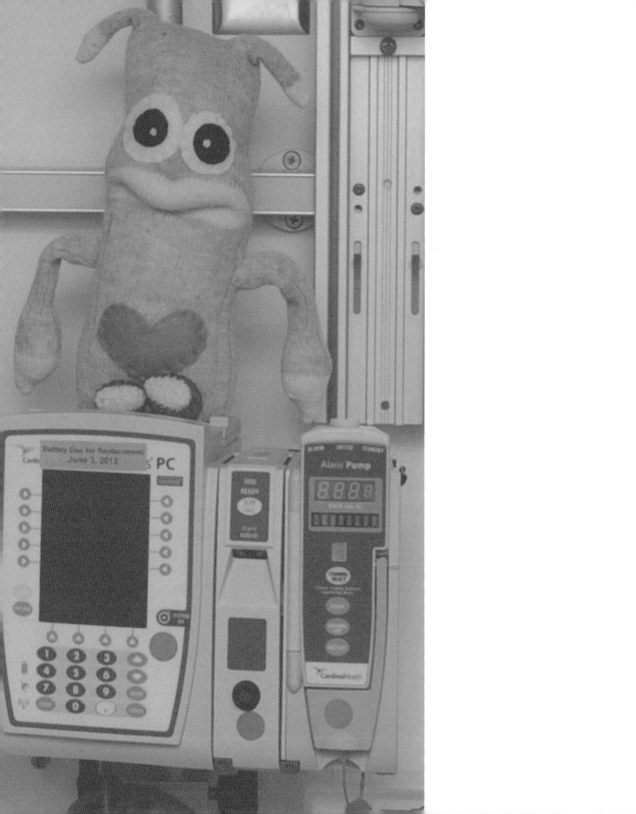

The other moms have decorated their areas with stuffed toys or little gifts. Some of the incubators have homemade quilts over top. It's nice. It makes things seem normal. I don't have anything like that but I asked my husband to bring some things from home this weekend.

Sometimes I feel down because all I can think about are all the things I've lost. It was always my dream to get pregnant and start a family. When I first became pregnant it was the happiest I'd been since my wedding.

I kept looking at my stomach in the mirror and thinking of how I would decorate the baby's room. We didn't have a lot of money, but I'm pretty handy and I painted the room a pretty yellow colour. I'd just bought some material for the bedding and curtains and was ready to start sewing, but then I had to go on bed rest. Now all of those things seem so meaningless. I just want my baby to get better so that we can go home and be a family.

I don't want to breastfeed. The nurses keep telling me that it's the best thing for the baby, but I just don't want to express milk. I know that breastfeeding is better than formula. I'm not stupid. All I ever dreamed of was breastfeeding my baby, but now I just feel too overwhelmed with everything that's going on.

Right now the baby is being fed through a feeding tube and later she can have formula. Lots of babies have formula and they do just fine. Claire said whatever decision I made had to be right for both me and my baby, but I still feel like some of the nurses and other moms are judging me—like I'm not doing what's best for the baby.

I feel judged a lot here in the NICU. Even Claire's husband Tom has asked

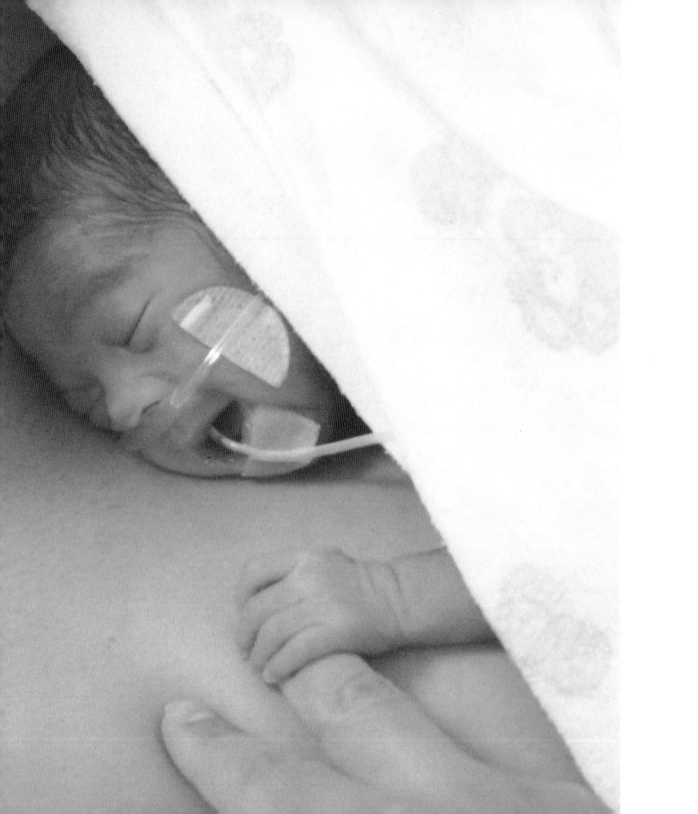

me why my husband isn't here with me. I told him that our business is just getting started and that it would go under if my husband wasn't back home, but I don't think he believes me.

There are some moms that spend a lot of time in the NICU and a lot who don't. I know that the baby furthest away from me only has his mom visit once a day between about six and eight at night. I talked to her the other day. Her husband left her two months before this baby was born and she has two other kids under five. She has no relatives in town and the only time she can come to the hospital is when her neighbour comes over to babysit. What else can she do?

※　※　※

I held my baby's hand today. It was the first time I felt like I could do it. She was so warm. The nurse showed me how to change her and I am going to try that later. She still has the breathing mask on but the nurse practitioner said that her lungs are getting stronger every day. She isn't strong enough to drink from a bottle yet, but maybe it won't be long.

I wonder if anyone ever expects to end up in the NICU? I sure didn't—even when I was on bed rest. I figured that if I did everything my doctor told me to do, I'd have a normal delivery.

I still remember when I went in for my prenatal appointment and my doctor told me that the baby's heart rate was lower than what it should have been. They put me in an ambulance and sent me here. All I could think of was that my baby was going to die. I just had a really bad feeling.

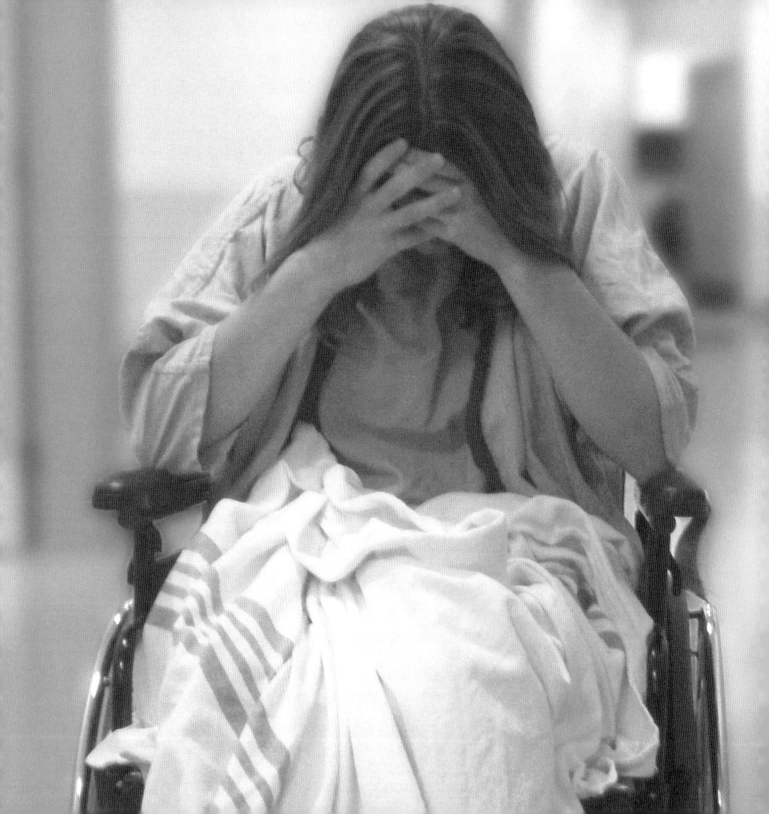

When I arrived here, they raced me in and hooked me up to the monitors. My baby's heart rate was half of what it was supposed to be. After that, everything seemed like a dream. Unreal. I remember lights and noises and horrible smells. Everything moved too quickly. Then everything went black when they put me to sleep for an emergency C-section.

My husband didn't make it for the delivery. He didn't even know where to find the hospital and then had a hard time finding the unit. As soon as he arrived, they took him to the NICU. I remember seeing him, but I was pretty out of it. I just wanted to know if we had a boy or girl and if our baby was alive.

When my husband finally came and told me that we had a girl and that she was alive, he looked scared. He's not used to babies or hospitals and I think it was too much for him. He'd never admit it, but I think he's relieved to go back to look after the business. I know he loves the baby, but I think that working hard to support us financially is his way of looking after our family.

🕸 🕸 🕸

"What's cerebral palsy?" I asked Claire. We were sitting in the coffee shop at the hospital. I'd only been here a week and I was already tired of the food. It was so expensive.

"I think it's an injury to the brain that affects nerves and muscles. Why do you ask?"

"Well the doctor told me this morning that my baby has been having some seizures and that may be a sign of her developing cerebral palsy later on."

Unexpected

"… it was terrifying… you don't know what to expect, you don't know what's gonna happen… everything they tell you is worst-case scenario so you're totally terrified - there's no other words to say it."

—Mother of a preterm baby

"Is he doing some tests?" Claire asked.

"I don't know. What kind of tests would he do?"

"I'm not sure," Claire said. "Talk to the nurse you like. She'll give you some information and help you figure out the right questions to ask."

"I'm a little worried." I pulled out my journal and checked it. "The doctor did say that seizures are not unusual in premature babies, but I just have a funny feeling about the whole thing."

"Trust your instincts," Claire said, "and ask for help. Remember when your baby was wet and you didn't know how to change the diaper? What did you do?"

"I went and asked the nurse to show me how to change it. She watched me do it the first few times until I felt comfortable."

"And now…"

"And now I can change her diaper whenever I need to." I felt happy just thinking about it. Changing a diaper was such a small thing, but it made me feel like a normal mother. It had been just so hard to do the first time.

"Okay. This is your baby, not the nurses' or the doctors' baby. She needs you to learn to speak up for her so she gets what she needs. Everyone who works here is great and they do a great job, but no one knows your baby as well as you. You're her mom."

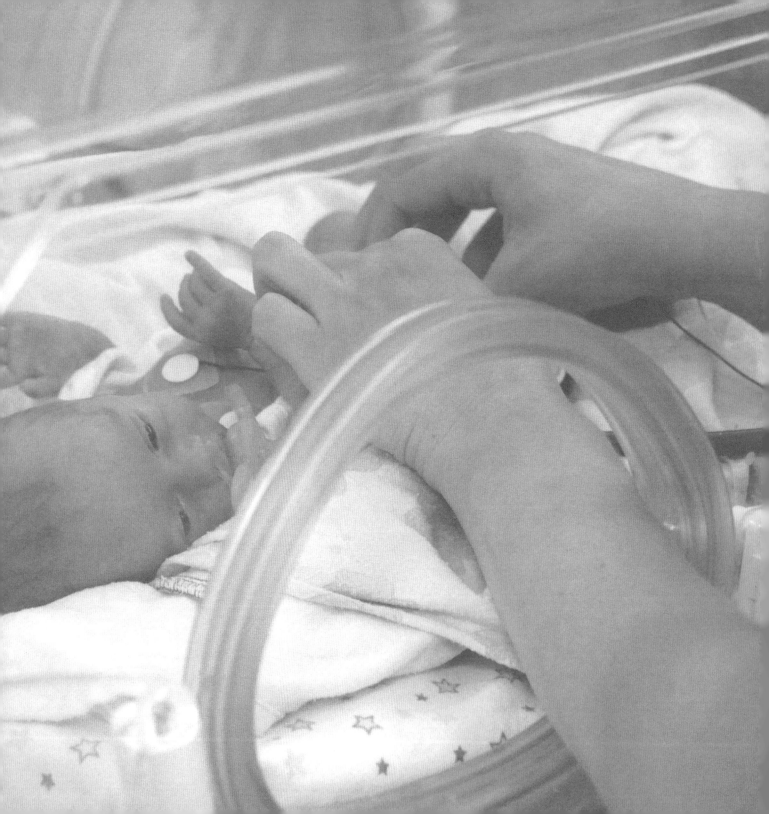

I could see where Claire was going with this. I had been in shock when I first saw my daughter in the NICU. Was it really just seven days ago? I had been content to have the NICU staff look after my baby because I was so overwhelmed. I've learned so much in just a week. I made a note in my journal to ask about the seizures.

Claire smiled at me. "When are you going to name that baby of yours anyway?"

⚘⚘⚘

I'm thinking of naming our daughter Claire Louise. I'm going to ask my husband tonight if that's okay. Louise was his mom's name and I think Claire was flattered that I wanted to name the baby after her.

I took Claire's advice and asked about the seizures. The doctor told me that there were many causes and that they would be doing some blood tests and possibly an EEG as well. When I asked him what that was, he took the time to explain exactly what the test would be like.

It's funny, I felt a little like a real mother when I diapered Claire Louise, but it was nothing like the feeling I got from taking control of my baby's health.

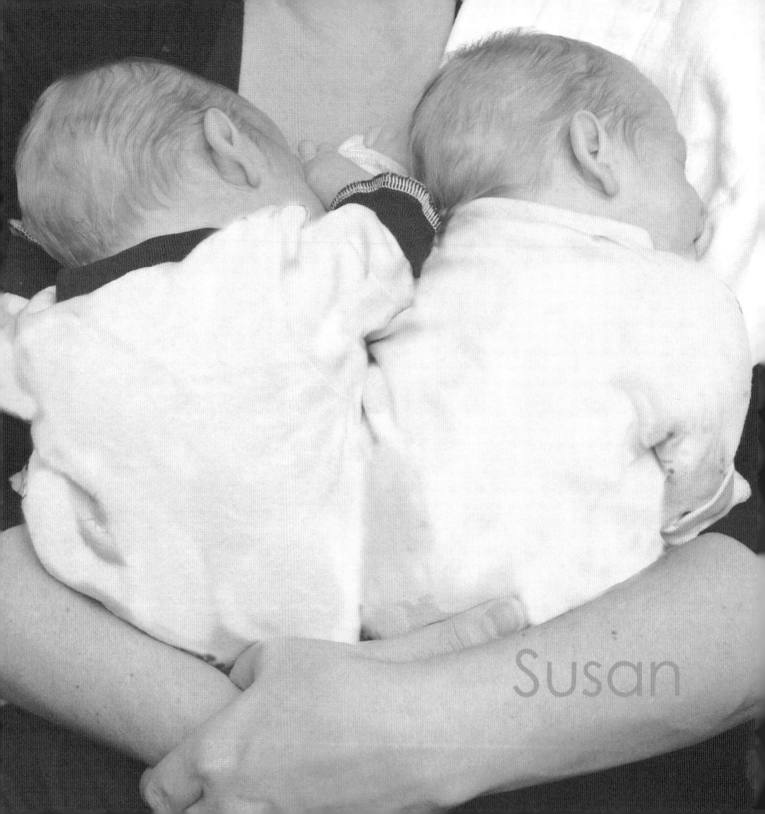

Susan

As a nurse working in the NICU, I had met many amazing parents—parents who had survived the ups and downs of watching their babies struggle for survival, sometimes thrive and sometimes die.

I thought I understood what they were going through, but I had no clue.

I gave birth to my twin daughters three weeks ago. I wanted to hold on until at least 28 weeks.

"Let's just make it to 28 weeks and you'll have a better chance," I kept telling the babies in my belly, but they had different plans. For me not having control was a huge issue. I felt completely helpless.

When the girls were born at 26 weeks, Jess was one pound, three ounces and Theresa one pound, eight ounces. From my work, I knew all of the stats about their chances of survival and knew all of the long-term problems they could face. Although I understood these things as a nurse, I had no clue what it was like to experience them as a mother.

It was surreal when the doctor told us that one of the girls might not survive. I remember seeing his lips move but I was concentrating on my breathing during labour and didn't hear what he said.

Unexpected

"[The nurse said] 'We're just gonna let nature take its course and when the baby is born you can hold her until she dies'. She didn't use the word 'dies' but that's basically what she was saying... I thought like, this is unbelievable, like how could this be happening? What did I do, what did my husband do,...why is this happening?"

—Mother of a preterm baby

"... she wasn't breathing very well, so they took her away, which was horrifying because, you know, you just have this baby and your intention is to hold it and bond with it afterwards and they take it away."

—Mother of a preterm baby

Finally I realized that he was asking if we wanted "compassionate care" to spare one of the twins from undue pain and suffering. How could I make that decision? I told him I wanted both babies. My husband told me later that I was yelling like a crazy woman at the doctor to keep both babies alive!

I was thrilled when I heard one baby cry and then the other. Then, the room was too quiet. Movements became urgent. I knew something was wrong.

I prayed for my babies to live and vowed to become a better person. I would give up everything I owned if only my babies would be allowed to live.

Then I waited… It was torture. I had some complications from the delivery and couldn't see the babies for 12 hours. My husband ran back and forth from the NICU with updates for me. He did his best, but I was frustrated because he couldn't give me the information I wanted. I kept sending him back to ask the right questions. Were they intubated or on CPAP? Did they have umbilical catheters? I knew there would be an IV and heart rate monitors, but I was desperate for details.

When I did finally see the twins, I cried. Jess looked very sick. I could see that she was struggling to survive. I noticed my colleagues watching me with concern but they kept their distance. I wasn't ready to talk to anyone. I just wanted to be with my husband and our babies.

I spent hours staring at my baby girls. I tried to remain positive, but the same thought ran through my head, *This wasn't the way it was supposed to be*. It was hard not to think that I—that we—deserved better than two sick babies delivered early.

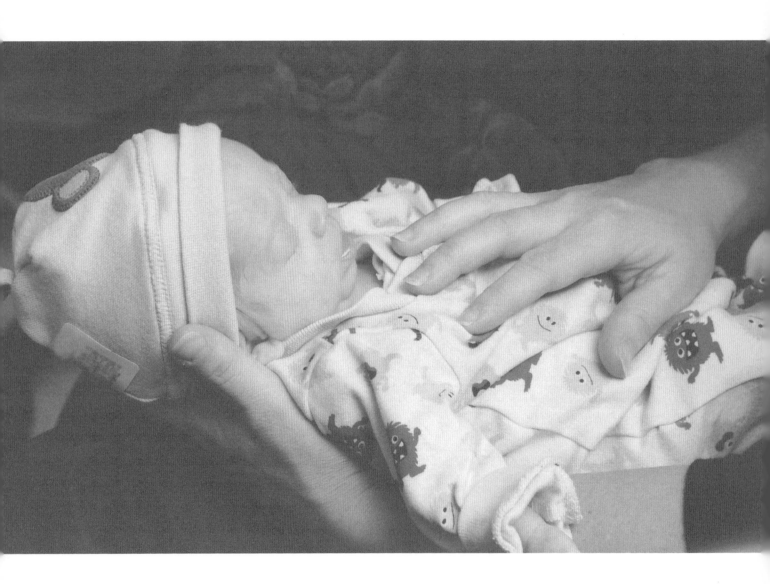

It took years for us to conceive. After three rounds of fertility treatments and two miscarriages, we became pregnant with twins. We actually celebrated when we made it past 10 weeks, then 16 weeks, then 26 weeks... I remember daydreaming about baby showers—about finally being the new mom in my circle of friends who already had children.

I wanted two healthy baby girls that I could cuddle and breastfeed and share with my mom and dad. My parents rarely come to the hospital to see the babies. My mom was here when they were born. I'll never forget the look on her face when she first saw them. It was a look of horror. I ended up comforting *her* while she sobbed about the loss of "normal" grandchildren.

I was tempted to tell her right then and there, "Mom, this is *my* normal." It has to be.

I am a very task-oriented person and I pride myself on being organized and efficient. When I became a mother in the very unit that I worked in, I felt like things were spiraling out of control. I knew how it worked from the other side—giving patient care and support, but I had no idea how to be on the receiving end—not knowing what came next. This new role of "mother" was filled with uncertainty and helplessness. How was I going to cope?

For the first few days I sat for hours watching the babies' chests rise and fall. Up and down. Up and down. I began expressing breast milk right away so that when they were strong enough to suckle, I would be able to feed them. I had some trouble at first and could have used some help, but I think, because I was a nurse, everyone thought I knew what to do.

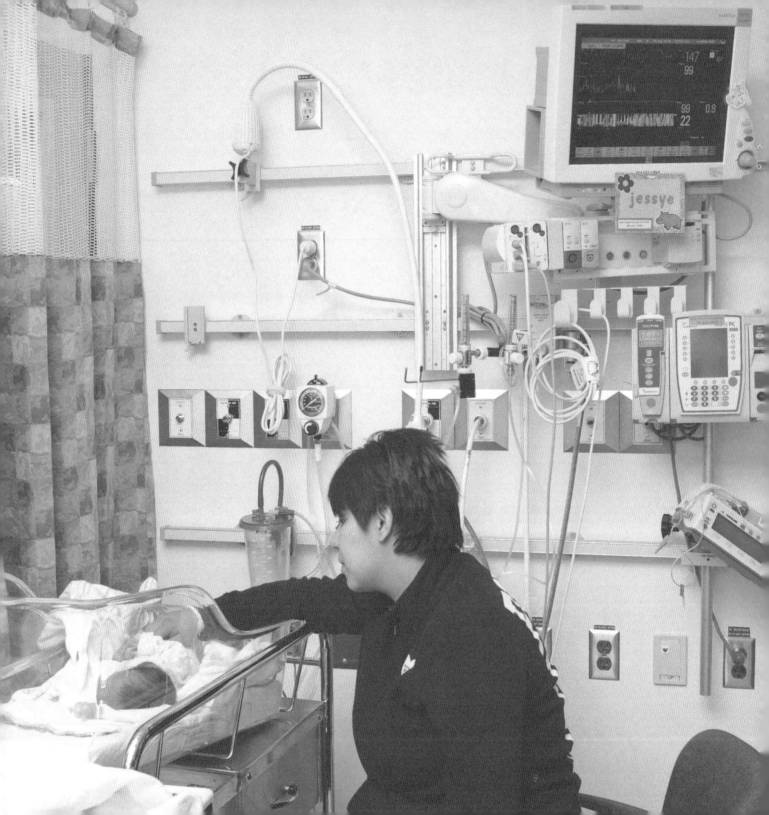

I spent lots of time in the breast pump room those first few days. It felt like the only thing I could do to nurture the babies was to express milk. The "Pump Room," as it was nicknamed, turned out to be a social gathering place of sorts. Over the next few days, I met other moms. Some had premature babies and others had full-term babies who were sick and had been admitted to the NICU for care.

The only thing we talked about was our babies and the stories we shared helped me get through a lot of the emotions I felt. There was a woman there, Claire, who had been in the NICU a while and we shared how we each coped with this life-changing event.

"I feel like I've lost control over my life," I told her.

"I think it's about acceptance," she said. "There are things you can control and things you can't. I had to let go of all my expectations of 'normal' and accept my new reality. Some days it's hard to find anything to be thankful for, but I try. Now I really appreciate when I can hold Matthew. I try to see each moment I spend with him as a gift instead of something I am entitled to."

"Even diaper changing?" another woman joked.

"Well maybe not that," Claire said with a smile. "One of my friends was due the same time I was and she had no complications. I found that so unfair. I couldn't even call and congratulate her. And then I felt guilty, so I eventually sent her a card."

"And it made you feel better?"

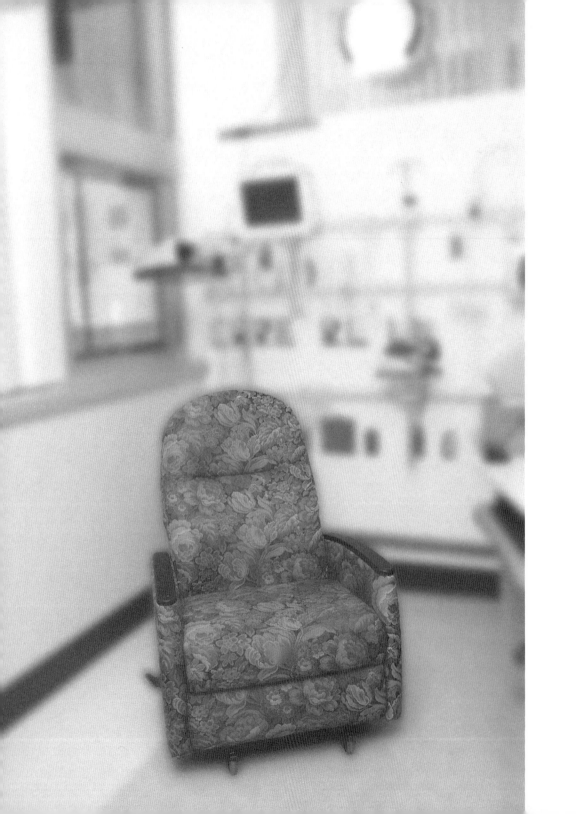

"No." Claire laughed. "But I decided to concentrate on what I *had* instead of what I *expected to have*. That gave me way more control over my situation.

"There is so much uncertainty in the NICU and things can change in a heartbeat. When I can do something—anything for Matthew I do it. Now I *can* feed Matthew and when I couldn't, I pumped and stored milk so that I could eventually feed him.

"The hardest part for me was to let go of the things I couldn't help him with. When he needed blood drawn, I couldn't take the pain of that pinprick away. When he needed an operation at another hospital, I couldn't control when he was transferred. It upset me that I couldn't, but there is a lot you just have to let go of when you have a sick child."

Claire's advice gave me a lot to think about.

It was awkward for me when some of the women shared stories about the way some nurses were treating their babies.

"Why did I have to have three nurses standing over me when I gave my baby his first real bath," one woman said. "They were all giving me advice, like they were afraid I was going to drown him. I was a nervous wreck. It should have been a great experience, but instead it was really stressful."

"I'm afraid to do anything with my baby," another woman said. I knew her name was Anna and that she spent a lot of time with Claire. She seemed to be having a really hard time. I often saw her crying as she sat by her baby. She was young and seemed lost and alone.

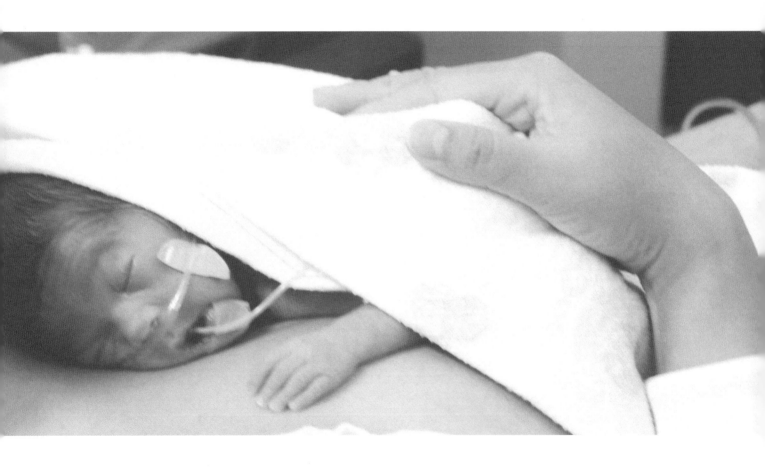

"Why don't you try to express milk for him," one of the women said.

Anna hugged her arms around her chest. "I don't want to," she said and began to cry.

"Everything's just so hard," she said.

"It will get easier," Claire said. "Today the nurse is going to show you how to do kangaroo care with your daughter."

Anna nodded. "I don't even really know what that is."

"Well, first you get comfortable on a chair and then the nurse will hand you your baby." I said.

"The baby goes skin-to-skin against your chest and you'll both be covered by a warm quilt."

Her eyes widened. "What about all the things attached to her?"

"They come along with her," I said, smiling. "Don't worry. The nurses will help you."

I felt for Anna. She was so anxious about everything. But I could see that the more information she had, the more relaxed she became. The other women and I talked about kangaroo care and gradually Anna's shoulders relaxed and she actually smiled.

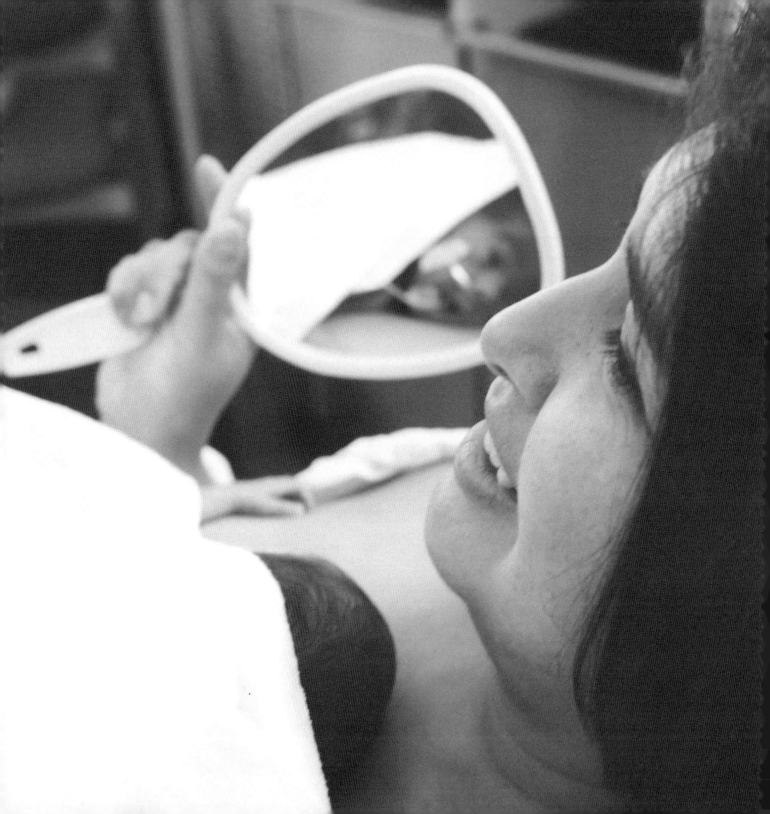

I hoped the other women wouldn't judge Anna too harshly for choosing not to breastfeed. Having a baby in the NICU is hard enough without being judged by others.

We all do the best we can. Some moms choose to breastfeed, some don't. Some want desperately to breastfeed and just can't produce enough milk. Not only do they feel guilty for not being able to provide milk for their baby, it's another loss they have to deal with. And then, some women produce enough milk to feed ten babies! The best end result, in my mind, is what's best for both the baby and the mother.

⁂ ⁂ ⁂

My babies were now being cared for on the same unit where I worked. This was really strange for me. I knew how I would do certain procedures and it was really hard to step away and watch other nurses doing things differently than I would do as a professional.

One of the problems with being an NICU nurse was that I knew everything that could go wrong and knew what to check. I spent most of the first few days watching the monitors instead of the babies.

As I constantly watched the monitors, I was judgmental when the nurses weren't quick enough to respond.

Are the babies breathing?

Are they eating?

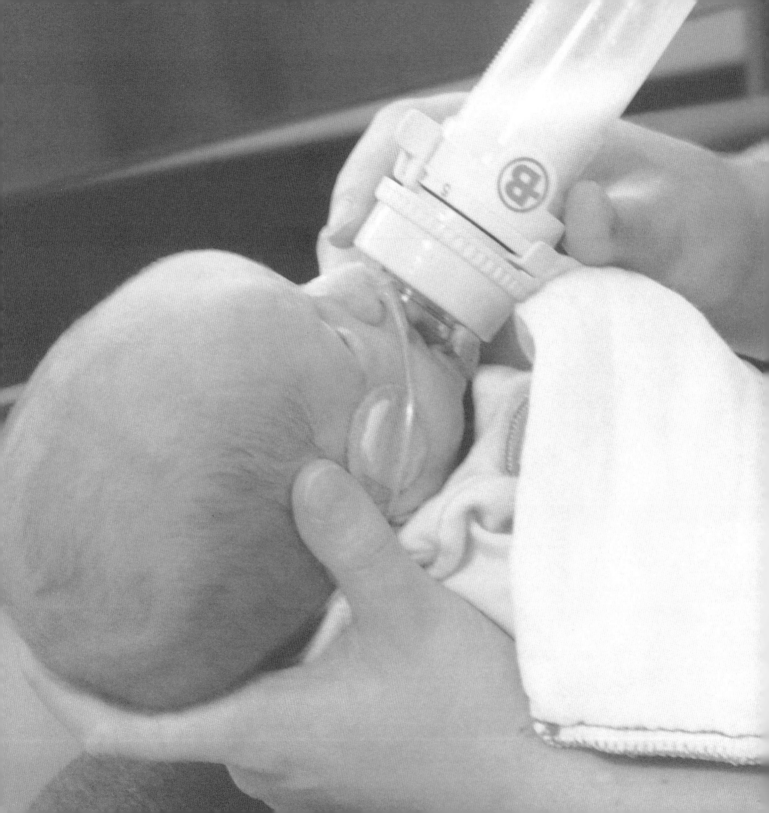

I think I was able to get through the first few days by focusing on *what* was being done rather than on my babies. I knew what all the machines did. I understood what the doctors told me. My twins both had jaundice and apnea that was treated with caffeine. They had anemia and required red blood cell transfusions. Jess had bradycardia or an abnormal slowing of her heart. The doctors couldn't figure out what was wrong. They didn't know what to tell me except that it was probably a heart defect.

I was really worried that both girls would have scarring to their lungs because they were born so early and that this would lead to further complications. The uncertainty of *not knowing* created so much anxiety that I stopped sleeping nights.

Soon I developed a routine. I began to enjoy my girls and each passing day it seemed like they were really going to pull through. I relaxed and was able to sleep more than a few hours a night. I did kangaroo care with Theresa for the first time. As I sat with her pressed to my chest, I could feel her heartbeat against me and I felt the tightness leave my body.

As I spent time with my daughters, I could see that even at a few days old they had different personalities. The more I focused on my babies, the less I noticed the machines and what others were doing around me. I began to let my colleagues do their jobs without hovering over every move they made.

Then, Jess developed an infection and the doctors couldn't determine the cause. She deteriorated rapidly and after nine days on this earth, my little girl died. I was devastated.

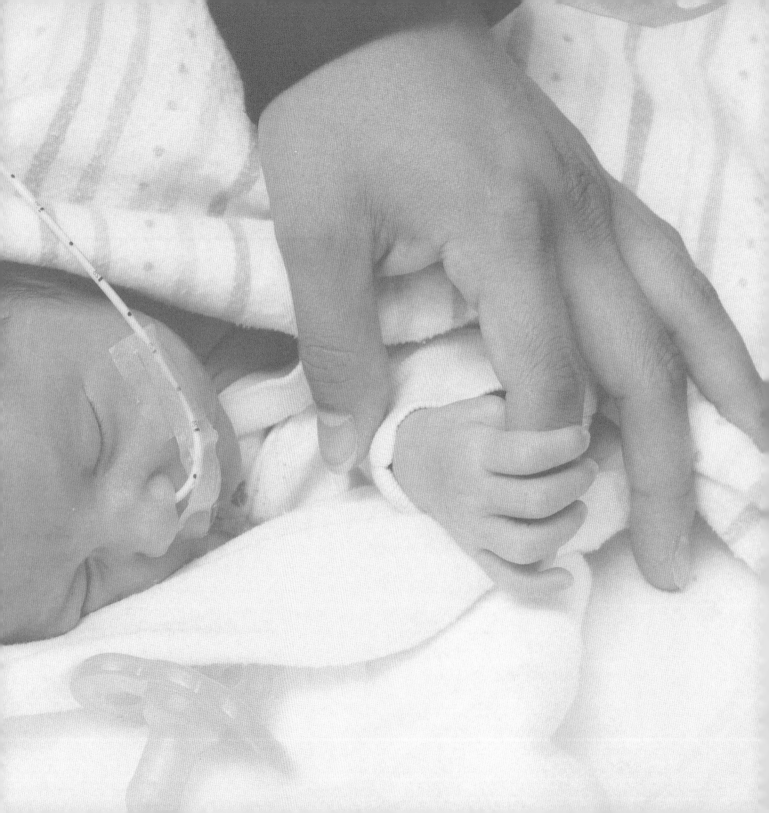

My husband and I had a photographer come and take photographs of each of us holding her little hands. Fortunately I was with her when she died. My husband wasn't and I think that he was more affected by this than he lets me know.

One of my colleagues asked if I wanted her to pack up Jess's things and I was thankful that I didn't have to do this myself. She put everything in a little box for us to take home. The social worker and someone from pastoral support helped us with arrangements.

Claire and Anna both gave me sympathy cards and I liked that. It made me feel like they understood that, even for her short life, Jess was a person—a human being.

When I told my family, they didn't really know how to respond. My mother told me that maybe it was better this way. I know that she didn't mean to hurt me, but she did. My parents did come to the memorial service we held for Jess, but I don't think they really understood why we had one.

I had seen other parents lose one of their twins in the NICU and it seemed that they dealt with the death one of two ways. Either they poured everything into the living twin and became over-vigilant—or they became very angry and looked for someone to blame.

The people they blamed were usually the staff—the nurses, doctors or nurse practitioners. Sometimes staff was moved to different parts of the unit to ease the parents' grief. This was hard on everyone. The staff often felt like they were being punished when they hadn't done anything wrong. The parents

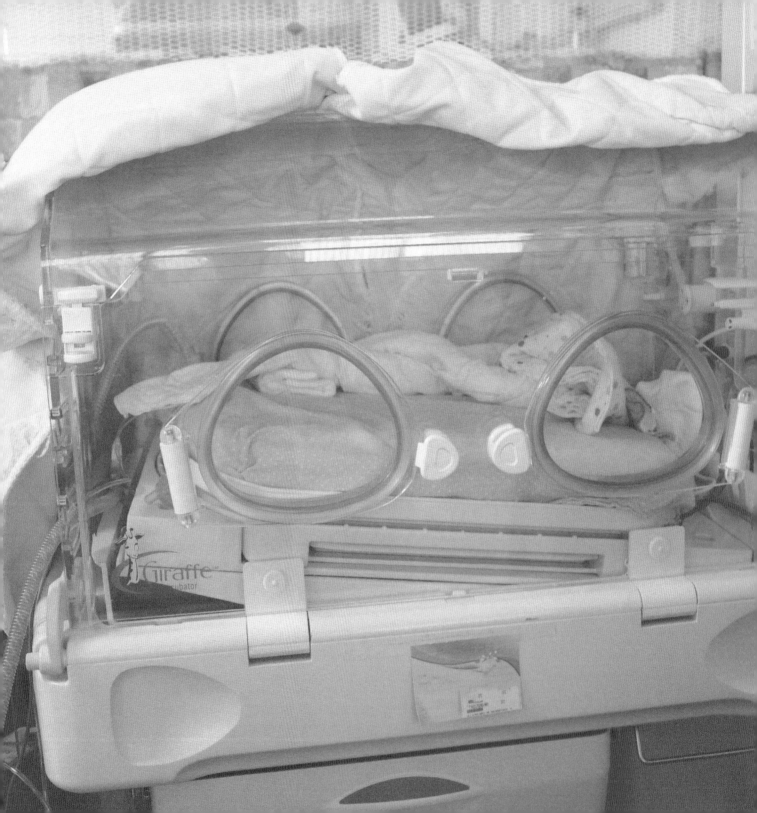

became bitter and sometimes anger became their focus instead of the surviving twin who so desperately needed them.

Having experienced the loss of a twin, I could understand both sides. Could things have been done differently in my daughter's care? Looking back, I can second and third guess every decision that was made. But there is no manual that comes with premature babies and each case is different.

During my years as a nurse, I had seen premature babies who seemed healthy, suddenly become very ill and die and I have also seen some miracles—babies who were given little chance of survival, not only survive but have no complications.

One of the hardest things to deal with regarding my daughter's death was that I still had a baby in the NICU. For the first few days, I found it difficult to leave the hospital even for a moment. I watched the monitors closer than ever and once, after a day of solid crying and countless more days of sleep deprivation, I blew up at a complete stranger—one of the relatives entering the pod.

The man walked in and strode right past the hand sanitizer. Why didn't he understand the importance of keeping a healthy and sanitized environment for these babies? An infection can mean life or death.

Claire came by today with her husband Tom. Matthew was in his brand new car seat. Tom was beaming with pride. They came to say good-bye. We exchanged emails and promised to keep in touch.

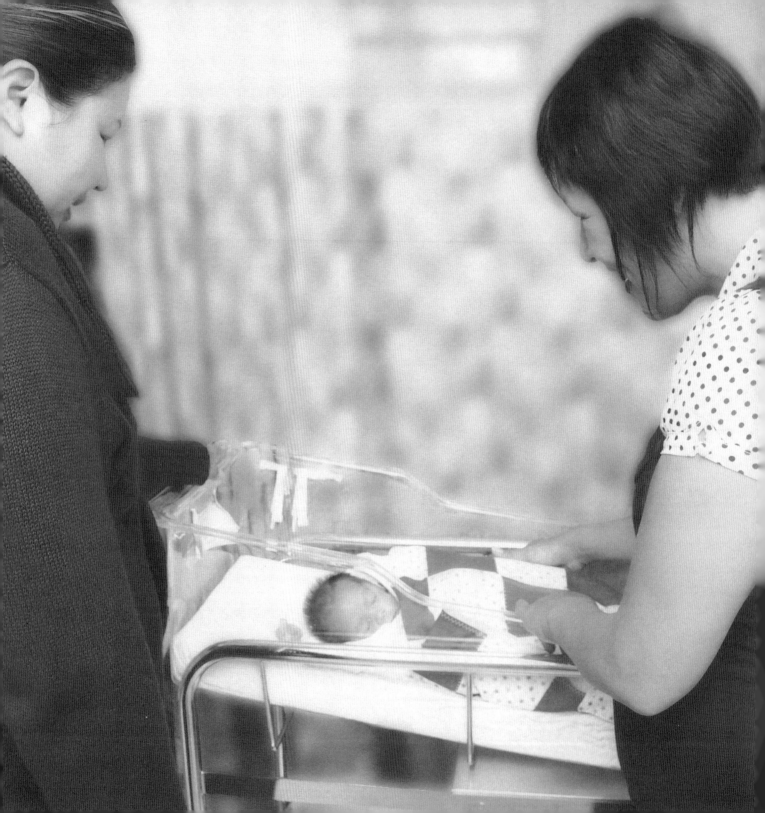

Anna's little Claire Louise is moving to the "feeder and grower" pod today. She will be just down the hall and we'll still be able to visit. Anna has changed so much. I remember her being so shy and reserved. As she developed relationships with the other moms, I saw her become more confident and assertive. She asks questions at rounds and the dark circles are almost gone from under her eyes.

I saw her talking with a teenage mom the other day. The teenager was awkwardly diapering her baby while Anna offered encouragement.

"You'll get through this," Anna told her. "I know everything seems strange right now. It's hard, but you can do it."

❧ ❧ ❧

Glossary

Acute Stress Disorder (ASD): A disorder caused by experiencing or witnessing a traumatic event. Symptoms can include appearing dazed, having flashbacks and experiencing anxiety, but disappear after a few weeks. ASD can develop into Post-traumatic Stress Disorder (PTSD).

Anemia: Decreased red blood cells or a reduced quantity of hemoglobin that can affect the distribution of oxygen to the organs in the body.

Apnea: Inability to breathe for longer than 15 seconds. Apnea is usually accompanied by bradycardia.

Bradycardia: A heartbeat that is slower than normal.

Breathing Mask: A plastic mask that covers the baby's mouth and nose for the delivery of air and/or oxygen.

Breathing Tube (Endotracheal Tube): A thin plastic tube that is inserted through the baby's mouth and into the trachea (windpipe) for the delivery of air and/or oxygen.

Cerebral Palsy (CP): A disorder of body movement that is caused by damage to, or abnormal development of the developing brain. CP can also include other physical and neurological abnormalities. There are many different types of CP.

Continuous Positive Airway Pressure (CPAP): The delivery of pressurized air (sometimes with additional oxygen) to keep the baby's lungs expanded during inhalation and exhalation.

Glossary

Electroencephalogram (EEG): Monitors and records electrical impulses of the brain to provide information about brain function.

Heart Rate Monitor: A machine that records information about the baby's heart rate. Monitors also record information about body temperature, respiration and blood pressure.

Hernia: Occurs when a portion of the intestine protrudes through a weak place in the abdominal wall. There are two types: inguinal and umbilical.

Intubate: To insert a tube into the trachea (windpipe) to allow air and/or oxygen to reach the lungs.

Intravenous (IV): Fluids, nutrition and/or medicine are delivered through a tube or needle inserted into the baby's vein.

Jaundice: A condition that makes the skin and whites of eyes look yellow. It is caused by a build up of bilirubin in the blood. Bilirubin is a chemical that is normally passed out of the body in urine and stool.

Kangaroo Care: A technique used with preterm babies in which the mother or father holds the baby skin-to-skin.

Nasogastric Tube: A flexible tube inserted through the nose or mouth to the stomach that is used to deliver nourishment. It is also used to remove fluid or air from the stomach.

Glossary

Neonatal Intensive Care Unit (NICU): An intensive care unit that specializes in the care of newborn premature or ill infants.

Pod: A room in the NICU that contains of several incubators or cots for a number of different babies. Different pods offer different levels of care depending on the baby's needs.

Post-traumatic Stress Disorder (PTSD): A severe anxiety disorder that can develop after witnessing or experiencing a traumatic event. Symptoms, including flashbacks, nightmares, anger and hypervigilance, last more than one month and cause decreased functioning.

Surfactant: A substance in the lungs that prevents the small air sacs (alveoli) from sticking together or collapsing. Often preterm babies have insufficient surfactant production and are given a surfactant to help with breathing.

Seizures: Seizures are caused by sudden abnormal activity in the brain. There are many different types and causes of seizures.

Umbilical Catheter: A small, flexible tube inserted into a blood vessel in the baby's navel. An umbilical catheter can be inserted into either a vein or artery. If it is inserted into a vein, it is used to give fluids and nutrition and to monitor blood pressure. If it is inserted into an artery, it is used to obtain blood samples, administer blood and medication and to monitor blood pressure.

Self Care Worksheet

It is easy to forget to look after yourself if you are experiencing a life-changing event. What are some of the things you can do to stay healthy?

- Eat several healthy small meals a day.
- Nap whenever you can.
- Go for a short walk outside—even if it is once around the block or to the corner store.
- Let go of events you can't control.
- Talk to someone who is supportive.

What helps you?

_____

_____

_____

_____

References

1. Landzelius KM. Charged artifacts and the detonation of liminality: teddy-bear diplomacy in the newborn incubator machine. J Material Culture 2001;6(3): 326.

Acknowledgements

Many people have been involved in the production of this book. Many thanks to the parents without whom this book would not have been possible.

We would also like to thank the following:

* The Neonatal Intensive Care Unit Family Advisory Care Team (NICU FACT) and the other health care providers who helped us understand the experience of preterm birth;

* Staff at the Royal Alexandra Hospital, Neonatal Intensive Care Unit;

* Julie Peter, BScN Honors Student, Faculty of Nursing, University of Alberta.

Made in the USA
Charleston, SC
17 April 2013